THE NEW CROHN'S FRIENDLY COOKBOOK

---

101 Delicious Recipes to Relieve Symptoms, Prevent Flare-Ups, and Boost Your Immune System - Includes a Complete Crohn's Nutrition Guide

Lydia Merrill

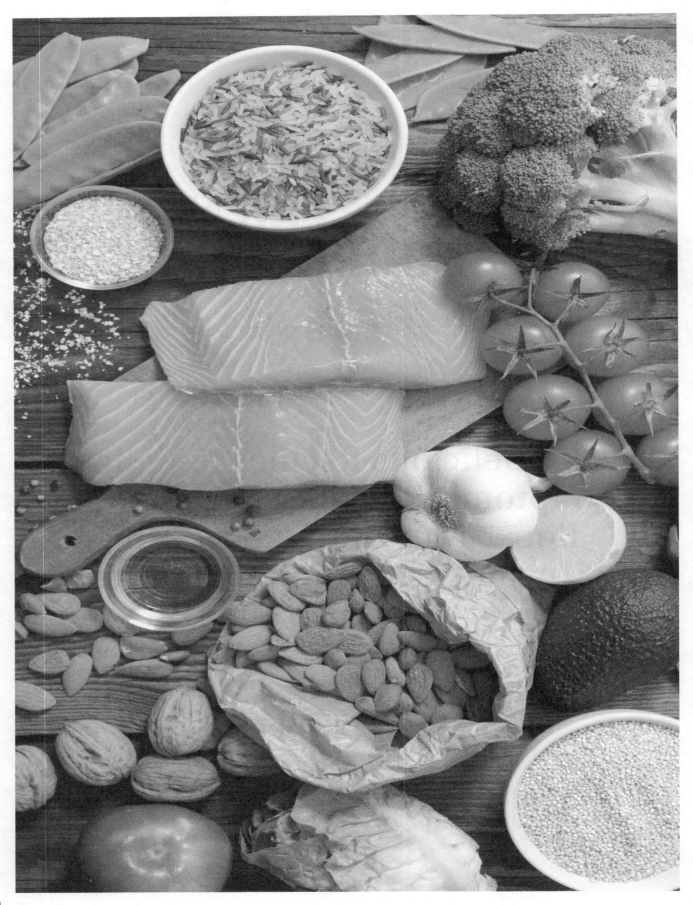

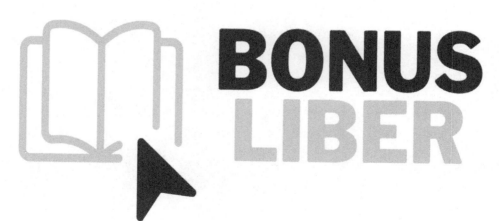

BONUS LIBER

Title: The New Crohn's Friendly Cookbook
Author: Lydia Merrill
Publisher: Bonus Liber Publishing
Website: www.bonusliber.com
Editors: James Peters, Carl Blackbirds
Cover: Designed by Getcovers
Interior Design: © Bonus Liber Publishing
Interior Photos: Bonus Liber Picture Archive, Freepix

ISBN: 9798731235372
First Edition: April 2021

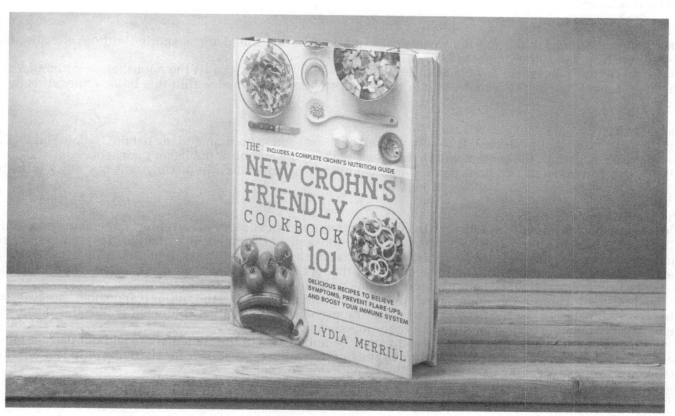

Table of contents

Breakfast

Pasta Dishes

Main Courses

Soups

Snacks

Dessert

CROHN'S DISEASE AND DIET

What is Crohn's disease?

Crohn's disease is a chronic, long-term condition where parts of the digestive system become inflamed. It's one type of condition called inflammatory bowel disease (IBD). According to the CCF (Crohn's & Colitis Foundation), as many as 780,000 Americans have this disease. Crohn's disease is most prevalent in the small intestine and the colon, but it can affect any part of your gastrointestinal tract (GI), from the mouth to the anus. Some sections of the GI tract may be involved, and other parts may be skipped.

Causes

While the precise causes of Crohn's disease are unknown, it is believed to be caused by a combination of environmental, immune, and bacterial factors in genetically susceptible individuals. Up to 20% of people with Crohn's disease also have a parent, infant, or sibling with the disease.

Symptoms

Symptoms of Crohn's illness frequently grow gradually. Some symptoms can also get worse over time. While it is likely, it is unusual for symptoms to progress abruptly and dramatically. Crohn's disease's early signs can include diarrhea, abdominal cramps, weight loss, fever, fatigue, feeling a frequent need for bowel movements, and blood in your stool. Sometimes, these signs can be mistaken for symptoms of another disease, such as food poisoning, stomach upset, or allergy. If any of these symptoms persist, you should see your doctor.

The symptoms can become more severe as the disease progresses. More troubling symptoms may include ulcers (they may occur anywhere from the mouth to the anus), a perianal fistula, shortness of breath or decreased ability to exercise (due to anemia), and inflammation of the joints and skin. Early detection and diagnosis will help you prevent serious complications and encourage you to start care early.

What Is a Crohn's Disease Diet Plan?

You've probably heard about various Crohn's disease diets. However, there is no scientifically validated diet for inflammatory bowel disease. Most experts believe that some patients, particularly during disease flares, can identify specific foods that trigger their gastrointestinal symptoms. You may notice that your gastrointestinal symptoms of gas, abdominal pain, bloating, cramping, and diarrhea are more controllable by avoiding your trigger foods. At the same time, you will give your irritated guts time to heal.

This is especially important if you are experiencing a flare-up of Crohn's disease symptoms. During a flare-up, spicy or greasy foods, whole grains, high-fiber fruits and vegetables, nuts and seeds, caffeine, and alcohol can all be taxing on your body.

If you have had absorbing nutrients issues due to Crohn's disease, it's vital to stick to a high-protein, high-calorie diet, even when you don't feel like eating. In this phase, an effective Crohn's disease diet plan, based on experts' recommendations, would put emphasis on eating regular meals -- plus an additional two or three snacks -- each day. This will help you get enough protein, calories, and nutrients. You will also need to take any vitamin and mineral supplements prescribed by your doctor. Only by doing so, you will be able to replenish the nutrients in your body by doing so.

What to Eat and What to Avoid

Food provides us with nutrients that provide energy and aid in the growth and repair of our bodies. Eating a healthy, balanced diet ensures that our bodies receive all of the nutrients they require. As we said before, the foods that induce Crohn's disease symptoms differ from person to person. Therefore, to know which foods to exclude from your diet plan, you must first determine which foods, if any, induce your symptoms. Once you've identified those foods, you can either avoid them or learn new ways to prepare them that will make them tolerable. To do so, you'll need to experiment with different foods and cooking methods to see what works best for you. For example, if certain raw vegetables cause a flare, you don't have to avoid them entirely. You may find that steaming, boiling, or stewing them will allow you to eat them without experiencing any adverse effects. If red meat causes fat in your stools, try ground sirloin to see if you can tolerate a leaner cut of beef. Alternatively, you could choose fish or low-fat poultry without skin as your primary protein source.

However, your diet may vary, depending on how active your Crohn's is. You may not be able to follow a balanced diet during a flare-up, but the principles summarized below are a good place to start when you're feeling well.

Fruit and vegetables

We should consume at least five portions of fruits and vegetables per day. Fresh, frozen, dried, or canned options are available. They're high in vitamins, minerals, and fiber, but you may need to limit your fiber intake if you have Crohn's disease. More information on fiber can be found later in this guide. If you have difficulty eating fruits and vegetables, such as having a stricture, your dietitian can help.

Starchy carbohydrates

These should account for slightly more than a third of the food we consume. They contain a lot of energy and nutrients. Breakfast cereals, pasta, bread, rice, and potatoes are examples of starchy foods. Some Crohn's patients may have difficulty digesting carbohydrates, resulting in symptoms such as bloating and diarrhea.

Protein

Proteins are required for both growth and repair. Poultry, lean meat, fish, beans, peas, and lentils are all excellent sources.

Dairy

Dairy foods, and alternatives like fortified soya milk, are the best source of calcium in the diet. They also provide protein and some vitamins. They include milk, cheese, yogurt and fromage frais. If you're allergic to milk, a dietitian can help you make sure you're getting enough calcium and vitamins in your diet.

Oils and spreads

Since they are high in energy, we only require a small amount. Remember that unsaturated fats, which are found in vegetable, rapeseed, olive, and sunflower oils, are healthier than saturated fats.

What about alcohol?

Alcoholics aren't completely off the table if you have Crohn's disease, but you need to practice moderation to ensure that you don't exacerbate your symptoms. According to some studies, people with Colitis who regularly consume large amounts of alcohol may be more likely to experience a flare-up.

How can diet help with my symptoms?

Making small changes to your diet may help you better control some common symptoms of Crohn's, such as loose and runny stools, bloating, wind, dehydration, constipation, weight loss, tiredness, nausea/vomiting and pain. While changing your diet can help you manage your symptoms, it doesn't replace the medical treatment suggested by your IBD team.

Loose and runny stools

Diarrhea, or loose and runny stools, is a common Crohn's symptom. Some people's diarrhea is unaffected by their diet. Others find that avoiding certain foods is beneficial. You could use a food diary to figure out which foods are causing your symptoms. Spicy or fatty foods, high fiber foods, gluten-containing foods, and dairy foods can all aggravate diarrhea. Caffeine, sweeteners, and alcohol-containing beverages can also worsen it.

Your dietitian can help you manage your diarrhea. They'll want to make sure you're getting enough nutrients and staying hydrated by eating and drinking enough. In some cases, they may suggest medications to help.

Dehydration

You can become dehydrated if your body does not have enough water. This can happen if you don't drink enough fluids or if your body loses too much fluid, such as when you have diarrhea or vomit.

Drinking water alone may not be enough to treat dehydration because your body has lost sugars and salts that must be replaced. You can buy rehydration solutions at pharmacies and supermarkets, but if you have kidney problems, you may be unable to use them. Some hospitals provide their own recipe for a homemade electrolyte mixture. Try adding salt to your food or eating a salty snack, such as crisps, with a glass of water or flat cola.

Drinking more water may increase your output and dehydrate you if you have a high-output ileostomy or a short bowel. Your doctor can advise you on whether you should limit your intake of ordinary fluids and instead use an electrolyte mixture. If you have a short bowel or are severely dehydrated, your IBD team may prescribe medication to slow the movement of your gut. It is essential to take this medication at the prescribed doses and times.

Bloating and wind

Bloating and wind can be caused by a variety of factors, including constipation, food intolerance, or swallowing air while eating or talking. Because no single solution works for everyone, it may take some time to find what works for you. Keeping a food diary can assist you in determining which foods are causing your symptoms.

You could try:

- eating when you're calm and relaxed, taking notice of what you eat and how much
- eating smaller meals, if you normally have large portions
- eating slowly, with your mouth closed
- chewing your food well to make it easier for your body to digest and absorb the nutrients
- avoiding fried, fatty or spicy food or food high in sugar.
- avoiding eating late at night

Constipation

If you have constipation, you will not pass stools as frequently as usual, and you may feel as if you are unable to completely empty your bowel. Your stools may be hard, lumpy, or dry, requiring you to strain on the toilet. You may also feel bloated and sick, and you may not want to eat much.

Constipation can be caused by rectum inflammation, a low fiber diet, not drinking enough fluids, and some medications, such as opioid pain relievers and iron supplements. You may experience constipation if you have an ostomy. Your stoma nurse or dietitian can assist you in selecting foods that will help you manage your stoma output.

These ideas may help you avoid or treat constipation:

- using a footstool, so your knees are higher than your hips when you sit on the toilet
- drinking more fluids to soften stools and make them easier to pass
- eating more fiber, but not if you have a stricture
- getting into a routine by trying to open your bowels at the same time of day for about 10-15 minutes, avoiding straining
- keeping active.

Laxatives that add bulk to the stools can help but aren't suitable for everyone. Speak to your doctor before taking any medicines for constipation.

Weight changes

Weight changes are common in people with Crohn's disease. If you eat less during a flare-up, you may lose weight and not get enough nutrients. Tell your doctor if you're losing weight without trying or if you don't feel like eating. You can help to keep your weight stable by:

- snacking between meals
- eating foods high in protein and calories
- having high-calorie drinks, like fruit milkshakes

On the other hand, taking steroids can make you want to eat more and cause you to gain weight. Be careful; being overweight can cause health problems, such as type 2 diabetes and heart disease. Exercise that makes you breathe faster, like swimming or jogging, can help you lose weight. Eating a balanced, healthy diet can also help.

However, it is critical not to restrict your dietary intake during a flare-up to avoid a lack of essential nutrients, so avoid dieting until your Crohn's is in remission. Measuring your body mass index and waist circumference can help you keep track of any weight changes.

You may be conflicted about losing weight during a flare-up. If you're trying to lose weight, you might feel good about your progress. However, you might be concerned about not eating a healthy diet. It's critical to consult with your doctor or a dietitian about any weight changes to ensure you're getting enough nutrients.

Tiredness

Many people with Crohn's disease experience extreme tiredness, known as fatigue. It's most common during flare-ups but also affects some people during remission. If you have anemia or suffer from anxiety or depression, you may be more prone to fatigue. Some medications can also make you feel tired.

Food may also play a role in your fatigue, especially if you aren't getting enough nutrients. See the previous section for more information on eating a healthy, balanced diet, and seek advice from your dietitian if necessary. If anemia is causing your fatigue, your doctor may advise you to take an iron supplement or eat more iron-rich foods. You could try eating five or six smaller meals throughout the day to help keep your energy levels up. Eating a light snack or drinking a milky or herbal caffeine-free drink before bed can help you avoid waking up hungry in the middle of the night.

Nausea and vomiting

Feeling and being sick - nausea and vomiting - is a possible Crohn's symptom. Some medications can cause nausea and vomiting. If you're taking methotrexate, an immunosuppressant, your doctor may prescribe folic acid to help with nausea and vomiting.

Here are some hints to help:

- eating something dry, such as white crackers or toast
- sipping a cold drink
- drinking ginger or peppermint tea
- eating foods containing ginger, like ginger biscuits
- avoiding eating too much or too quickly
- avoiding fried, greasy or strong-smelling food
- avoiding drinking large amounts of fluid.

Which nutrients are essential in Crohn's?

Vitamins and minerals

Your body requires vitamins and minerals to work and remain healthy. Your Crohn's disease may make it difficult for you to absorb enough vitamins and minerals from food. Iron, vitamin D, vitamin B12, and calcium, for example, may not be properly absorbed.

Eating a healthy, balanced diet may help your body's vitamin and mineral levels. If blood tests reveal that you have low vitamin and mineral levels, your doctor may advise you to take supplements to restore your vitamin and mineral levels. Also, if you suspect you may be lacking in any of these nutrients, consult your doctor or dietitian.

Iron

Iron deficiency is common in people with Crohn's disease. A lack of iron in the diet, blood loss, and problems absorbing iron from food are all possible causes. Anemia, which occurs when fewer red blood cells carry oxygen around the body, can be caused by a lack of iron.

Common symptoms of anemia include:

- feeling tired and lacking in energy
- fast or irregular heartbeat
- feeling short of breath
- pale skin.

If your diet is low in iron, your dietitian may advise you to eat more iron-rich foods. These include green, leafy vegetables, eggs, cereals and bread with added iron (fortified), meat and pulses like peas, lentils and beans. It's harder for the body to absorb and use iron from non-meat foods, but having some vitamin C at the same meal can help. You could, for example, drink a glass of orange juice with your fortified breakfast cereal. Drinking a lot of coffee or tea can also make it more difficult for your body to absorb iron from food.

Vitamin B12

Usually, you get enough vitamin B12 from your diet. It can be found in foods such as meat, fish, milk, cheese, eggs, and some breakfast cereals fortified with vitamin B12. If you eat a vegan diet, you may not get enough of this vitamin and may need to supplement it.

Vitamin B12 is absorbed in the terminal ileum, the last section of the small intestine. You may not be able to absorb vitamin B12 if you have surgery to remove the ileum or if there is inflammation in that area. This can result in low vitamin B12 levels in the body, making you tired. Your doctor may prescribe B12 injections every three months to keep your B12 levels from falling too low.

Vitamin D

When your skin is exposed to sunlight, your body produces vitamin D. It's also found in egg yolks, oily fish and foods fortified with vitamin D, such as margarine and breakfast cereals.

People who have Crohn's disease are at risk of having low vitamin D levels. If this is not treated, you may develop bone pain. Recent research suggests that you may be more prone to flare-ups, but it's unclear whether low vitamin D levels cause flare-ups or are the result of flare-ups.

Calcium

Calcium is essential for healthy bones and teeth. Calcium can be obtained from dairy products, fish with bones – such as sardines – and calcium-fortified foods such as breakfast cereal and bread. If you cannot consume dairy products, you may be deficient in calcium, and your doctor may prescribe calcium supplements. Lactose intolerance is discussed further below. If you are receiving steroid treatment, you may need to take calcium and vitamin D supplements. Steroids have been linked to an increased risk of bone thinning over time.

Fiber

Fiber is a carbohydrate found in plants that is digested in the colon. It aids in the bowel's maintenance by softening and bulking up stools, making them easier to pass. Dietary fiber is essential for good health. It can help you maintain healthy levels of cholesterol, blood pressure, and weight. It can also aid in the treatment and prevention of constipation.

People who have Crohn's disease may be more sensitive to the effects of fiber in the gut. Fiber can help some people reduce symptoms during a flare-up and stay in remission. On the other hand, fiber can aggravate some people's symptoms. If your Crohn's disease is in remission but you still have symptoms like abdominal pain, constipation, and diarrhea, reducing your fiber intake may help.

It's critical to consult with a dietitian before changing your fiber intake to avoid missing out on the health benefits. For example, they may advise some people to cut back on fiber for a short period during a flare-up before gradually reintroducing it into their diet.

Fiber-rich foods include:

- starchy foods, such as porridge, oat bran, high-fiber breakfast cereals, potato with the skin on, wholemeal or wholegrain bread and pasta
- peas, beans and pulses, such as baked beans, lentils, chickpeas
- fruit and vegetables
- nuts and seeds.

Healthy adults should eat 30g of fiber each day. Children under 16 need between 15g and 25g, depending on their age. If you're trying to eat more fiber, increase the amount gradually to avoid wind, bloating, and stomach cramps. Since fiber attracts water, it's important to drink eight to ten cups of fluid daily to avoid getting dehydrated. Water, herbal teas, and milk are healthier than sugary or fizzy drinks. If you've had strictures (narrowing your intestine) or blockage episodes, your dietitian may recommend a low-fiber diet. This is to avoid fiber getting stuck in narrow parts of the bowel, which may increase the risk of a blockage.

Low-fiber foods include:
- tinned fruit in juice with no skin, pith or seeds
- fleshy parts of vegetables with no skin or seeds
- sieved tomatoes and tomato sauces
- fruit juices – one serving a day
- processed breakfast cereals like cornflakes and puffed rice
- white pasta, bread and rice.

Lactose intolerance

Lactose is a sugar found in dairy products, such as milk, cheese and cream. An enzyme in the gut, called lactase, breaks down lactose so the body can absorb it. If you're lactose intolerant, your body doesn't produce enough lactase. This can cause:

- bloating
- wind
- stomach rumbling and pain
- nausea – feeling sick
- diarrhea – loose and runny stools.

People with Crohn's have the same risk of being lactose intolerant as the general population. But if you have Crohn's in your small bowel, you're more likely to be lactose intolerant. Some people with Crohn's only get symptoms of lactose intolerance during a flare-up. Following a low-lactose or lactose-free diet may help you control your symptoms. You can choose lactose-free dairy products - try to buy ones that are fortified with calcium. Read the labels carefully on pre-prepared foods, as some have lactose added.

Small amounts of lactose, such as a bit of milk in your coffee, may be digestible. Checking the ingredients list will give you an idea of how much lactose a product contains. If lactose is near the bottom of the list, it means there is only a trace of it in the product.

Lactose intolerance symptoms are similar to flare-ups, so seek advice from your doctor before eliminating lactose. He can also make sure you're getting enough calcium and vitamins in your diet, both of which are essential for bone health. If you have been diagnosed with lactose intolerance, you should be tested again in the future because lactose tolerance can change over time.

Gluten

Some people with Crohn's disease may also have a condition called celiac disease. It means that you cannot digest a type of protein called gluten, which is found in wheat, rye, and barley. Some of the symptoms of celiac and IBD overlap, such as bloating, abdominal pain and diarrhea.

If you don't have celiac disease but get symptoms when you eat gluten foods, you may have a sensitivity to wheat, rye or barley. Some people with Crohn's have symptoms of irritable bowel syndrome (IBS). The low FODMAP diet limits wheat, rye and barley and may relieve IBS symptoms. Of course, it's important to consult with a dietitian before starting this diet.

If you suspect you have celiac disease or a sensitivity to wheat, barley, or rye, consult your doctor or a dietitian before changing your diet. It is crucial to obtain a diagnosis so that you can receive the appropriate monitoring and treatment. Before you can be tested for coeliac disease, you must consume gluten. Also, if you avoid gluten-containing foods, you may not get enough fiber in your diet.

Is a Low-Residue Diet a Crohn's Treatment Diet?

A low-residue diet is one that is low in specific foods that contribute to stool residue. Many people with Crohn's small intestine disease have a narrowing or stricture of the lower small intestine (the ileum). A low-fiber, low-residue diet can help them reduce abdominal pain, cramping, and diarrhea. While scientific evidence is lacking, this diet may help some people reduce the frequency of their bowel movements. On a low-residue diet, you should avoid the following foods:

- Raw fruits and vegetables
- Corn hulls
- Seeds
- Nuts

Can Keeping a Daily Food Diary Help Me Manage My Crohn's Disease?

Yes. Keeping track of the foods you eat on a daily basis can assist you in identifying "offenders" – foods that may trigger symptoms. Avoiding these foods may help you control your symptoms, especially if your disease is active. A daily food diary can also help your doctor determine if you're getting a well-balanced diet. It can tell you if you're getting enough protein, carbs, fats, and water. It can also tell you if you're getting enough calories to keep your weight and energy levels stable.

To begin your diary, keep a small notebook in which you record the foods you eat each day as well as the serving sizes. In the notebook, write down the date, the food, and any symptoms you experienced after eating it. After a month or two, set up a time with a registered dietitian to review your food diary. The dietitian can determine whether you're getting enough essential nutrients from a well-balanced diet or if you need supplements. Proper nutrition aids in the healing of the body and keeps you healthy. Having a nutrition discussion with a dietitian is therefore essential for your overall health and Crohn's disease management.

2 WEEKS MEAL PLAN

WEEK #1

Weekday	Breakfast	Lunch	Dinner	Snack / Dessert
Sunday	Chia Pudding with Papaya	Grilled Salmon Skewers with Fennel and Tomato Salsa	Eggplant Casserole with Mozzarella	Smoothie with Mango, Banana and Carrot
Monday	Banana Shake with Cottage Cheese	Zucchini Carpaccio with Basil and Ricotta Dumplings	Carrot Curry Soup + Couscous with Chicken	Smoothie with Avocado and Pears
Tuesday	Fruity Breakfast Quark	Indian Vegetable Spiced Rice with Mango Chutney	Tamarind Chicken Skewers with Avocado and Tomato Salad	Strawberry Cake with Lime and Buttermilk Cream
Wednesday	Colorful Oat Breakfast	Herb Omelet with Smoked Salmon	Green Beans au Gratin on Spelt Semolina	Tuna Muffins
Thursday	Green Spoon Smoothie with Papaya	Tagliatelle with Radicchio in Creamy Ham Sauce	Zucchini Soup + Vegetable Sushi with Nori Seaweed	Millet Pancakes
Friday	Crunchy Granola	Thai Crab Salad served in the Papaya	Sheep Cheese Pasta	Avocado Crostini with Goat Cheese and Tomatoes
Saturday	Carrot and Apple Porridge with Cinnamon	Indian Style Soy Strips	Brazilian Fish Pot with Coconut and Chili	Baked Figs with Cream Cheese and Pistacchio Filling

WEEK #2

Weekday	Breakfast	Lunch	Dinner	Snack / Dessert
Sunday	Chia Coconut Pudding	Asian Noodle Soup	Baked Chicken Breast with Spinach and Sheep Cheese	Strawberry Papaya Drink with Kiwi Puree
Monday	Granola with Banana	Tuna Pasta in Spicy Tomato Sauce	Hawaiian Curry Soup + Salmon and Spinach Roll	Chocolate Raspberry Slices
Tuesday	Cereal Porridge	Vegetable Schnitzel in an Almond Crust with Smoked Salmon	Rocket and Radicchio salad with Grapefruit and Scallops	Smoothie with Spinach and Strawberries
Wednesday	Fruity Carrot Salad with Cream Cheese Bread	Hearty Semolina Slices with Paprika Vegetables	Salmon Cutlet on Kohlrabi Salad with Fennel and Watercress	Energy Balls
Thursday	Multigrain Porridge with Baked Peach	Italian Bean and Tuna Salad with Celery and Tomatoes	Stewed Cucumbers with Salmon and Dill	Apple and Majoram Breads with Leek
Friday	Cottage Cheese Breakfast	Pumpkin Soup with Ginger + Bulgur Salad	Pollock Fillet with Romanesco and Olives	Pineapple and Cucumber Salsa with Spring Onions
Saturday	Almond Pancakes with Blueberries	Watercress and Cucumber Salad with Smoked Salmon	Fortifying Broth + Carrot Tagliatelle and Pine Nuts	Banana Berry Smoothie with Grapefruit

Breakfast

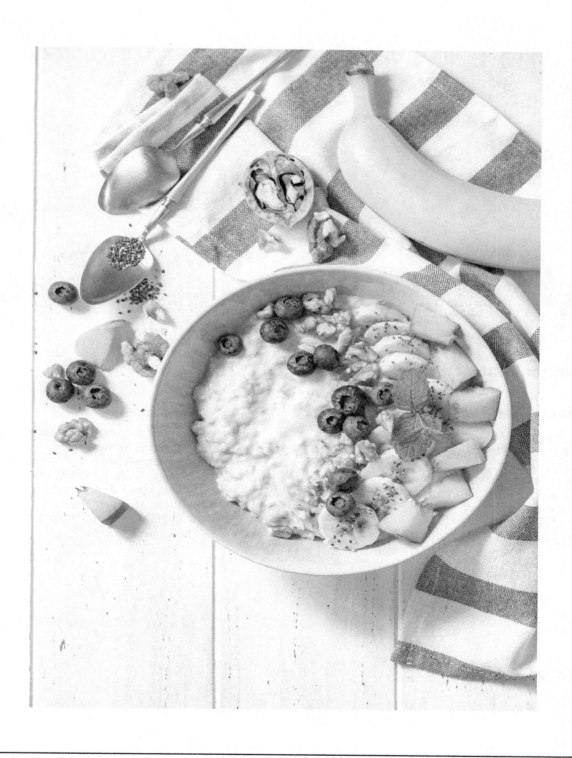

Colorful Oat Breakfast

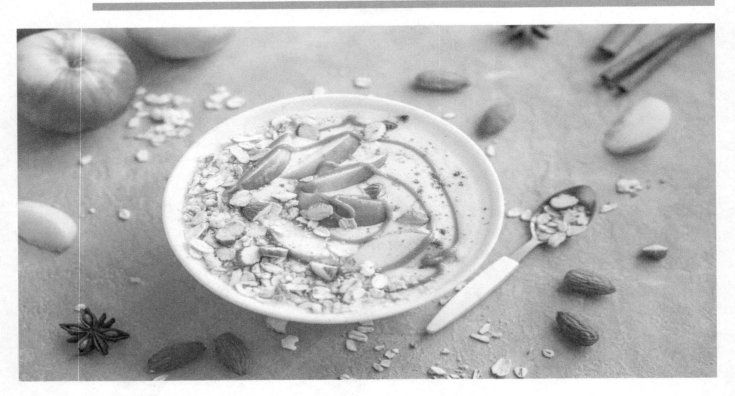

Preparation Time: 10 mins

Ingredients per person:

- 1 small (approx. 100 g) apple
- 1 large (approx. 100 g) carrot
- some lemon juices
- 50 g crunchy oat flakes
- 150 g (1.5% fat) natural yogurt
- 1 teaspoon of linseed oil
- 1 pinch of cinnamon
- 1 pinch of cayenne pepper

1. Wash the apple, quarter, core and grate with the skin, peel and grate the carrot.
2. Add a splash of lemon juice.
3. Mix the raw vegetables with the oat flakes, yogurt, linseed oil and the spices - done.
4. sh of lemon juice.
5. Mix the raw vegetables with the oat flakes, yoghurt, linseed oil and the spices - done.

Nutritional Value

394 Kcal	11 g Fat	59g Carbs	13g Protein	10 g Fiber

Colorful Fruity Carrot Salad with Whole Meal Cream Cheese Bread

Preparation Time: 30 mins

Ingredients for 2 people:

- *200 g Carrots*
- *200 g Natural yogurt*
- *1 tsp Walnut oil*
- *200 g pineapple*
- *30 g chopped walnuts*
- *30 g Desiccated coconut*
- *2 slices fine whole meal bread*
- *50 g grained cream cheese*

1. Peel the carrots and cut them into coarse strips with a vegetable slicer. Put in a salad bowl and mix with the walnut oil. Grab the pineapple by the leaf, peel, cut out the stalk and cut the pulp into small pieces.
2. Lightly toast the chopped walnuts and desiccated coconut in a coated pan without adding any fat until it starts to smell. Add the mixture to the carrots along with the pineapple pieces. Stir the yogurt until smooth and mix it into the salad. Let everything sit in the refrigerator for about 30 minutes.
3. Spread the cream cheese on whole meal bread slices and serve with the salad.

Nutritional Value per Serving

466 Kcal	25 g Fat	43g Carbs	15g Protein	11 g Fiber

Banana Shake with Cottage Cheese

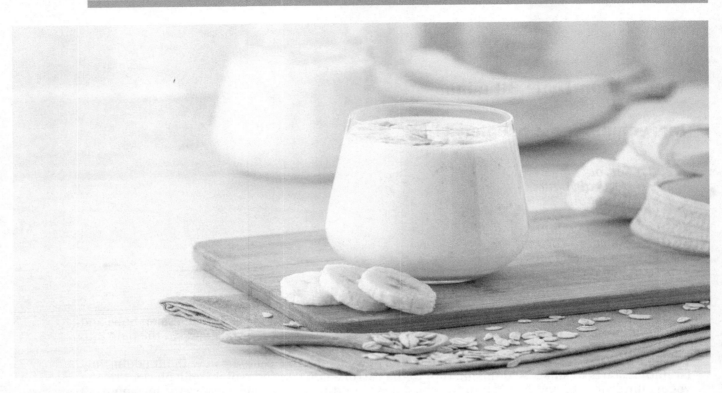

Preparation Time: 10 mins

Ingredients for 1 serving

- *1 banana*
- *100 ml Oat milk*
- *100 g Quar*

1. Put all ingredients in a blender or mixing bowl and mix or puree finely.
2. Pour into a glass and serve immediately.

Nutritional Value per Serving

187 Kcal	2g Fat	26g Carbs	11g Protein	2g Fiber	2 BE

Fruity Breakfast Quark

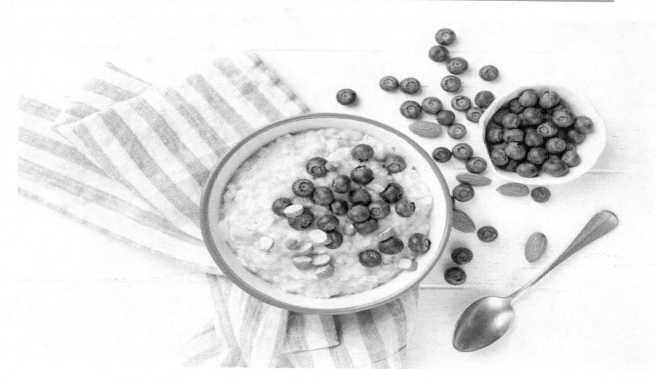

Preparation Time: 10 mins

Ingredients for 1 Serving

- *3 tbsp fresh milk*
- *3 tbsp low-fat quark*
- *1 tbsp linseed oil*
- *1 tbsp wheat germ oil*
- *if you like: 1 teaspoon honey*
- *1 squirt of lemon juice*
- *1 handful of fresh fruit*
- *to taste: almond slivers or nuts*

1. Mix all ingredients, including washed, selected fruit, in a blender and pour into a bowl.
2. Sprinkle with sliced almonds, chopped walnuts or lightly roasted hazelnuts as desired.

Nutritional Value per Serving

407 Kcal	24g Fat	31g Carbs	16g Protein	3g Fiber

Multigrain Porridge with Baked Peach

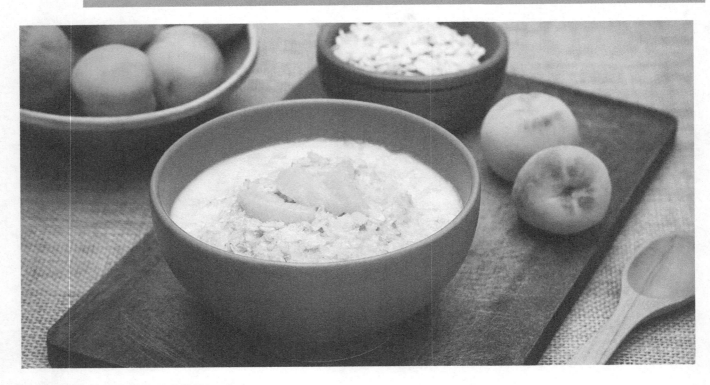

Preparation Time: 25 mins

Ingredients for 2 people:

- *2 peaches*
- *4 tbsp*
- *maple syrup*
- *5-grain flakes*
- *400 ml milk (1.5% fat)*
- *salt*
- *1 tsp cinnamon*

1. Wash the peaches, cut in half, stone them and place the halves in a baking dish with the opening facing up.
2. Pour 1-2 teaspoons of maple syrup into each peach half and bake the peaches on the oven shelf in a preheated oven at 200 ° C (fan oven: 180 ° C, gas: level 3) for 15–20 minutes.
3. In the meantime, put the cereal flakes, milk and a pinch of salt in a saucepan and bring to a boil over medium heat, stirring constantly. Let simmer for 1 more minute.
4. Stir cinnamon into the porridge, remove from heat and cover with cling film or a lid and leave to soak for 5 minutes.
5. Divide the porridge between bowls. Place the baked awl halves on the porridge. If the porridge is too thick, just mix in some milk.

Nutritional Value per Serving

374 Kcal	9 g Fat	58g Carbs	12g Protein	5g Fiber	15g Added Sugar

Almond Pancakes with Coconut and Cinnamon Curd

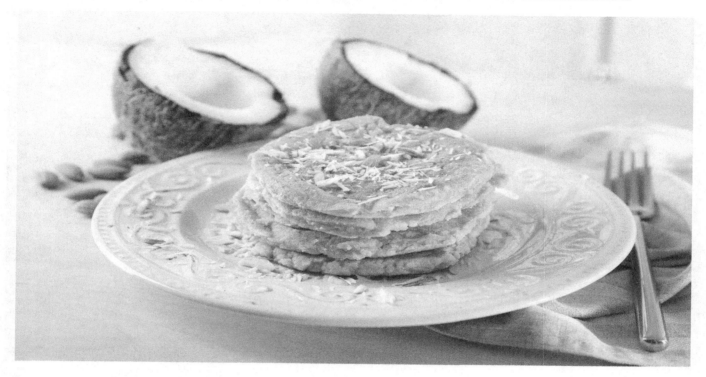

Preparation Time: 20 mins

Ingredients for 2 peolpe

- 2 eggs
- 6 tbsp (90 ml) milk
- 50 g ground white almonds
- 5 tsp (15 g) flaxseed flour
- Vanilla powder
- cinnamon
- 1/2 teaspoon baking powder

Ingredients for the quark:

- 300 g cream quark
- 100 ml coconut milk
- 2 tbsp linseed oil
- 4 tbsp desiccated coconut
- 2 teaspoons of cinnamon

Nutritional Value per Serving

620 Kcal	53 g Fat	8g Carbs	26g Protein	6g Fiber

1. Mix the eggs in a bowl with the milk and a pinch of salt with a whisk.
2. Then add the almond flour and flaxseed flour as well as a pinch of vanilla and cinnamon each and mix in very thoroughly.
3. Gradually add 4 tablespoons of water. Let the dough soak for 10 minutes.
4. After swelling, mix the baking powder into the batter.
5. Heat a little oil in each pan and fry several pancakes one after the other.
6. Keep the finished pancakes warm on a plate.

1. In a large bowl, stir the cream curd with coconut milk and linseed oil until smooth. Then season with desiccated coconut and cinnamon.
2. Serve with the pancakes and garnish with coconut chips if you like.

Tip: *The pancakes are gluten free. The flaxseed flour provides additional binding - it is also great for homemade bread, pastries or simply as an ingredient in muesli.*

Chia Coconut Pudding

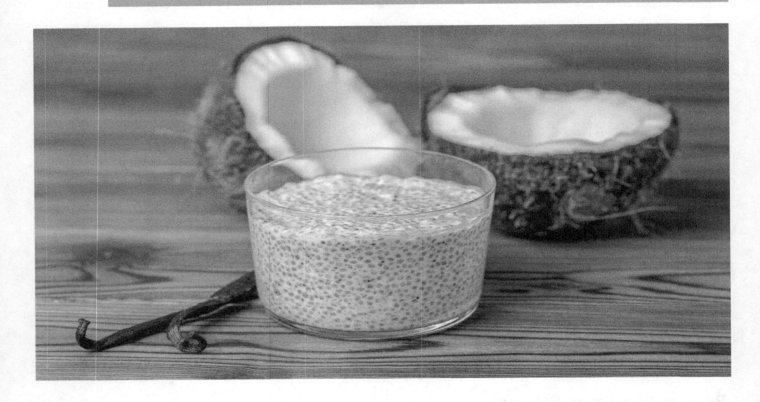

Preparation Time: 20 mins

Ingredients for 2 people:

- 30 g chia seeds
- 100ml coconut milk
- 1 teaspoon virgin coconut oil or rapeseed oil
- 2 tbsp desiccated coconut
- 2 tbsp wholegrain spelt flakes
- 0.25 l of water
- 1 teaspoon rice syrup

1. Mix the chia seeds with coconut milk and 1/8 l water and leave to soak for 10 minutes.
2. Then stir everything again and cover and let the mixture soak in the refrigerator for 12 hours - preferably overnight.

Variation 1: with whole meal spelt flakes and berries

Preparation Time: 60 mins

- *1 teaspoon of virgin coconut or rapeseed oil*
- *2 tbsp desiccated coconut*
- *2 tbsp wholegrain spelt flakes*
- *1 teaspoon rice syrup*
- *100 g (of your choice, also TKI) berries*

1. The next day, heat the oil in a non-stick pan and roast the coconut flakes and spelt flakes over medium heat for 3 to 4 minutes while stirring until golden brown.
2. Drizzle with the rice syrup, mix well and remove from heat.
3. Sort the berries (e.g., strawberries, blueberries, raspberries or currants), wash them, pat dry, and, if necessary, cut them into small pieces.
4. Take the chia pudding out of the refrigerator, stir again and layer with the coconut flake mixture and the berries in large glasses or bowls.
5. Finish with a few berries and serve immediately.

Nutritional Value per Serving

408 Kcal	28g Fat	26g Carbs	12g Protein	14g Fiber	3 BE

Variant 2: with apple and sprouts topping

Preparation Time: 60 mins

- *0.5 apple*
- *1 handful of blueberries*
- *30 g almonds*
- *2 tbsp radish or alfalfa sprouts*

1. The next day wash the apple, remove the stem and seeds, chop it up. Wash the blueberries and pat dry. Spread the apple, blueberries, almonds and sprouts on top of the chia coconut mash for serving.

Nutritional Value per Serving

241 Kcal	16g Fat	9g Carbs	8g Protein	8g Fiber	0,8 BE

Oat or Spelt Porridge with Nuts

Preparation Time: 10 mins

Ingredients for 2 people:

- *6 tbsp (60 g) oat or spelt flakes*
- *½ l (1.5% fat) milk*
- *alternatively: ½ l oat drink or other vegetable milk*
- *50 g coarsely chopped, possibly soaked almonds*
- *to taste: low-acid fruit*
- *1 pinch of cinnamon*
- *1 pinch of turmeric*

1. Stir oat or spelt flakes into the milk or, alternatively, the plant milk and bring to a boil.
2. Cook for 2 minutes while stirring, then add the almonds (if the intestine is sensitive, soak the almonds overnight).
3. Bring to the boil again briefly and allow for swelling for about 10 minutes.
4. Mash ½ a banana or grate 1 apple, add to the still-hot porridge, and then sprinkle with the spices.

Nutritional Value for preparation with cow's milk (per serving). with fruit

400 Kcal	25 g Fat	30g Carbs	16g Protein	

Nutritional Value for the praparation with oat drink(per serving) with fruit

372 Kcal	19 g Fat	38g Carbs	12g Protein	8g Fiber

Nutritional Value for preparation with cow's milk (per serving). without fruit:

374 Kcal	19 g Fat	31g Carbs	19g Protein	6g Dietary Fiber

Nutritional Value for the praparation with oat drink(per serving) without fruit

351 Kcal	19 g Fat	34g Carbs	12g Protein	7g Fiber

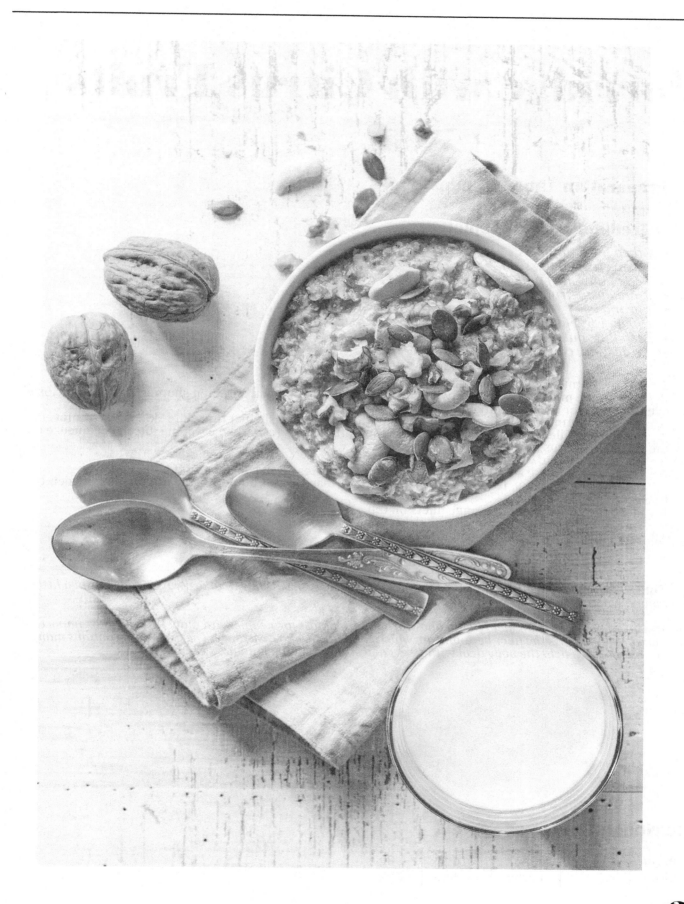

Porridge with Citrus Fruits

Preparation Time: 10 mins

Ingredients for 2 people:

- *4 tbsp fine oat flakes*
- *4 tbsp crushed flaxseed*
- *0.25 l (1.5% fat) milk*
- *1 pink grapefruit*
- *1 orange*
- *150 g (1.5% fat) natural yogurt*
- *2 tsp Pine nuts*
- *for dusting: cinnamon powder*

1. Mix the oatmeal with the flaxseed in a saucepan.
2. Pour in the milk and 100 ml of water, bring everything to a boil and then simmer with the lid closed over low heat for 6 to 8 minutes, stirring occasionally.
3. In the meantime, peel the grapefruit and orange so generously that the white skin is also removed.
4. Cut out the fillets between the individual separating skins (catch the escaping juice and squeeze out the rest of the citrus fruits well).
5. Stir the juice into the oatmeal.
6. Cover the porridge and let it soak for another 5 minutes on the switched-off hotplate.
7. Remove the porridge from the stove, mix with 1 teaspoon of liquid honey and divide between two bowls.
8. Place the grapefruit and orange fillets on top.
9. Spread the yogurt over it and sprinkle with the pine nuts.
10. Serve dusted with a bit of cinnamon.

Tip: *The porridge solidifies when it cools and is therefore also suitable to take away. Simply stir in a little boiling water to warm up.*

Oatmeal *porridge is an ideal filling and warming breakfast for people with diabetes. The most important ingredient in oats is the fiber beta-glucan, which combats insulin resistance. The grain also contains many B vitamins, which help the body deal with stress and strengthen the immune system.*

Nutritional Value per Serving

360 Kcal	14 g Fat	36g Carbs	16g Protein	8g Fiber

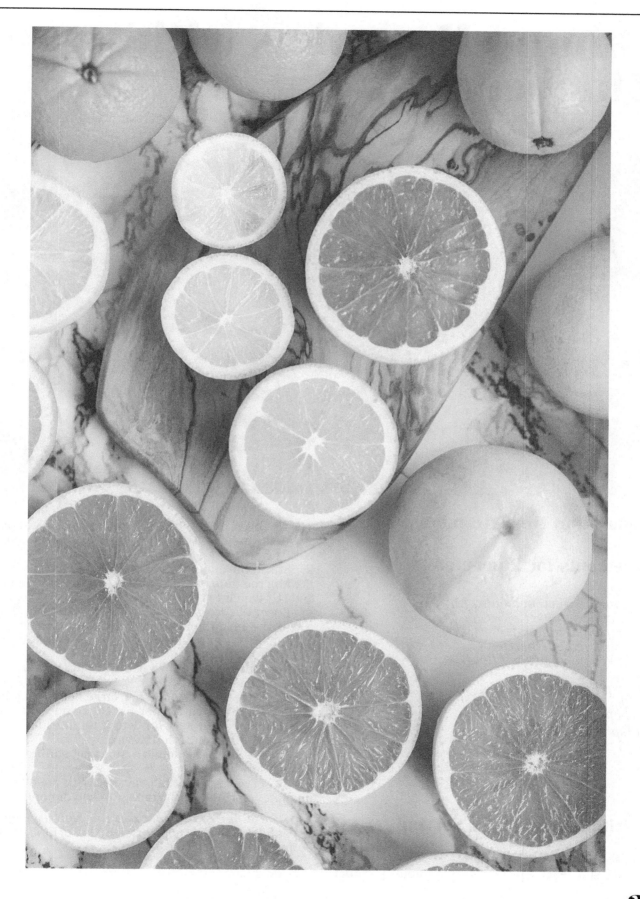

Almond Pancakes with Blueberries

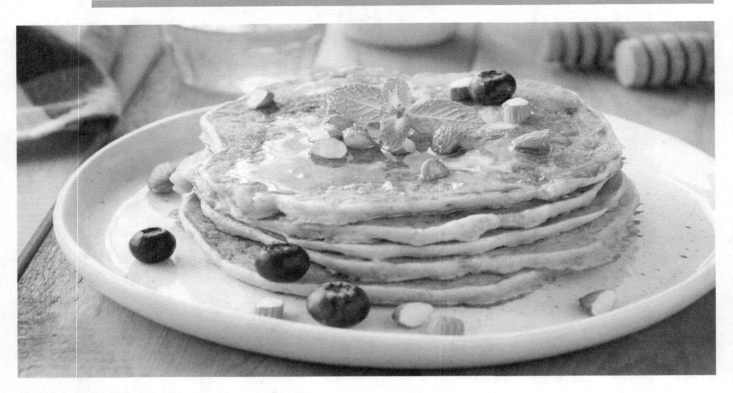

Preparation Time: 18 mins

Ingredients for 2 people:

- 2 Eggs
- 100 ml unsweetened oat drink
- Raw cane sugar
- 30 g ground almonds
- 1 tbsp dried blueberries
- 60 g Whole meal spelt flour
- salt
- 0.5 tsp baking powder
- 150 g (fresh or frozen) blueberries
- tbsp Flaked almonds
- 1 Tsp virgin coconut oil
- 0.25 tsp Cinnamon powder

1. The eggs with the oat drink - soy drink should be avoided - as well as whisk the sugar in a mixing bowl with a whisk.
2. Stir in the almonds and dried blueberries.
3. Mix the flour, a pinch of salt and the baking powder and stir well into the egg mixture.
4. Cover the dough and let it soak for about 15 minutes.
5. In the meantime, wash the fresh blueberries, sort them and pat dry (allow frozen food to thaw in good time).
6. Toast the almonds in a pan without fat over medium heat. Take out and let cool.
7. Heat 2 teaspoons of oil in a large non-stick pan. Add 2 tablespoons of batter per pancake and bake on each side over medium heat for 1 to 2 minutes until golden brown. Take out and keep warm.
8. Process all of the dough in this way, adding a little oil if necessary.
9. To serve, arrange the pancakes with the blueberries on plates, sprinkle with cinnamon and almonds.

Tip: *These fluffy little pancakes are high in fiber and a sweet filwler. Drizzle with 1 tablespoon of liquid honey as desired.*

Nutritional Value per Serving

440 Kcal	23g Fat	33g Carbs	18g Protein	10 g Fiber

Chia Pudding with Papaya

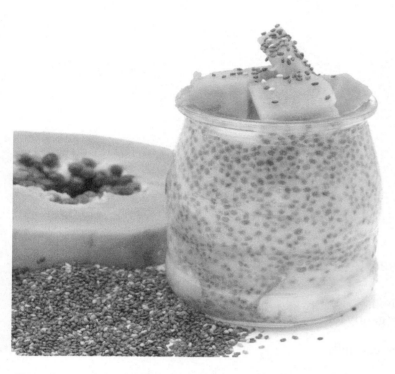

Preparation Time: 10 mins

Ingredients for 1 person:

- *20 g Chia seeds*
- *70 ml Rice milk*
- *alternatively: oat milk*
- *1 papaya*
- *1 splash Lemon juice*
- *1 tbsp linseed oil*
- *2 tbsp chopped walnuts*
- *alternatively: almonds or cashew nuts*

1. Put the chia seeds in a bowl and add the milk - they should be well covered because the seeds bind a lot of liquid.
2. Stir, set aside and let soak for at least 1 hour, preferably overnight, in the refrigerator.
3. Peel the papaya and remove the seeds.
4. Drizzle with lemon juice and cut into small cubes.
5. Mix together with the linseed oil into the chia pudding. Sprinkle with the nuts.

Nutritional Value

460 Kcal	34 g Fat	29g Carbs	11g Protein	14 g Fiber

Quinoa Breakfast Porridge with Strawberries

Preparation Time: 10 mins

Ingredients per person:

- *200 ml of water*
- *100 ml lactose-free milk*
- *alternatively: 100 ml water*
- *1 teaspoon of sugar*
- *140 g quinoa*
- *1 pinch of salt*
- *200 g strawberries*
- *5 stalks of fresh mint*
- *2 tbsp almond slivers*
- *½ teaspoon cinnamon*
- *as desired: maple syrup or cinnamon sugar*

1. Bring the water and milk with sugar to a boil.
2. Add quinoa and a pinch of salt and simmer gently for 5-8 minutes until the liquid is absorbed.
3. In the meantime, wash the strawberries carefully and cut them into bite-sized pieces.
4. Wash the mint, shake dry, chop finely and mix with the strawberries.
5. Remove the porridge from the heat, fold in the almond slivers and cinnamon with a wooden spoon.
6. Pour into small bowls, pour the strawberries over them and sweeten with maple syrup or cinnamon sugar as desired.

Nutritional Value per Serving

395 Kcal	12g Fat	58g Carbs	13g Protein	8 g Fiber

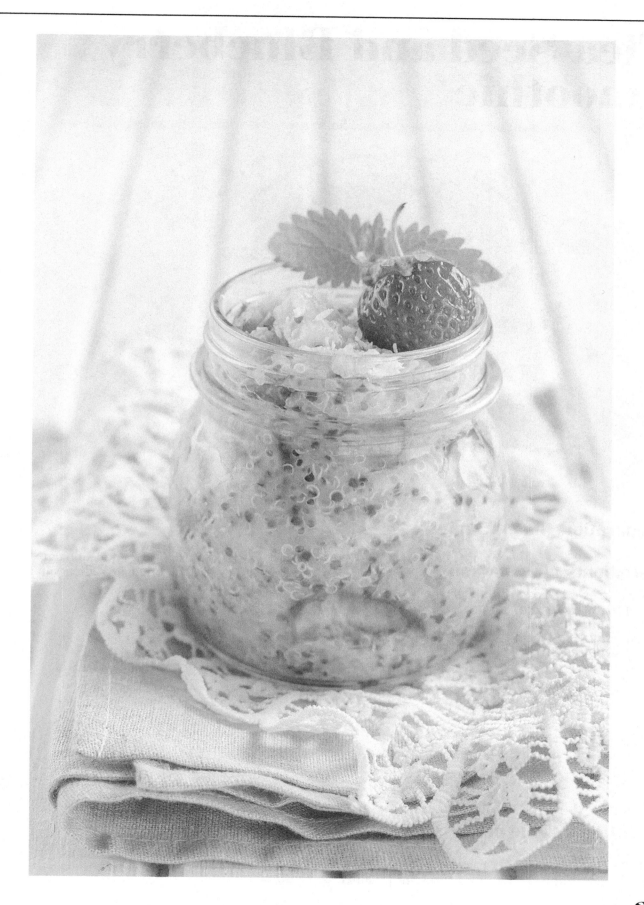

Flea Seed and Blueberry Smoothie

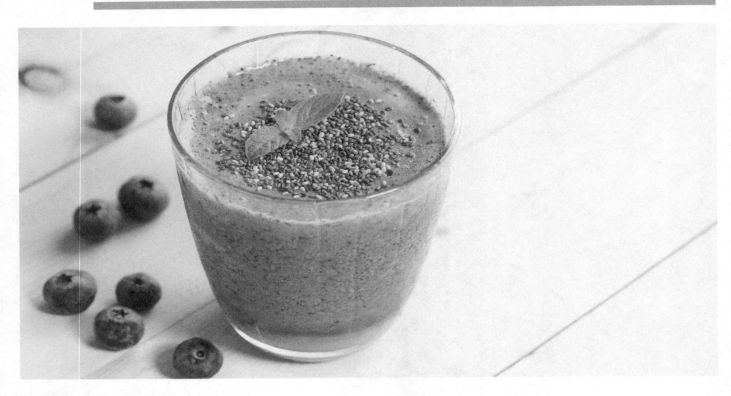

Preparation Time: 15 mins

Ingredients for 1 person:

- *100 g (fresh or frozen) blueberries*
- *50 g (fresh or frozen) spinach*
- *100 ml Coconut milk*
- *1 tsp Flea seeds*
- *1 tsp Chia seeds*
- *1 tsp linseed*

1. First, wash the fresh berries and spinach.
2. Put together with all other ingredients in a blender and whisk into a smoothie.

Nutritional Value per Serving

113 Kcal	5 g Fat	11g Carbs	5g Protein	12 g Fiber	0,9 BE

Granola (Crunchy Muesli) with Banana

Preparation Time: 30 mins

Ingredients for 12 servings (approx. 600 g):

- *2 ripe bananas*
- *4 tbsp coconut oil*
- *1 teaspoon ground vanilla*
- *1 teaspoon cinnamon*
- *2 pinches of salt*
- *100 g sunflower seeds*
- *50 g puffed amaranth*
- *200 g flaked almonds*
- *50 g desiccated coconut*
- *100 g crispy gluten-free oat flakes*
- *alternatively: spelt flakes*

1. Pre heat the oven to 180 degrees Celsius.
2. Line a baking sheet with parchment paper.
3. Peel and roughly dice the bananas.
4. Puree the oil, vanilla and salt in a tall mixing beaker with a hand blender.
5. Mix the sunflower seeds, amaranth, almonds, desiccated coconut and oat flakes in a bowl.
6. Add the banana puree with a wooden spoon and mix well.
7. Spread the mixture evenly on the baking sheet and bake in the oven on the lower rack for 25-30 minutes.
8. Mix well every 8 minutes so that the granola browns evenly.
9. Take the granola out of the oven and let it cool completely on the tray. Then fill it into a tightly fitting jar or glass for storage.
10. To serve, fill approx. 50 g granola per person into bowls. For example, serve with around 200 g (vegan) yogurt and 125 g raspberries or blueberries.

Nutritional Value per serving (50g)

255 Kcal	18 g Fat	15g Carbs	8g Protein	4 g Fiber

Green Spoon Smoothie with Papaya

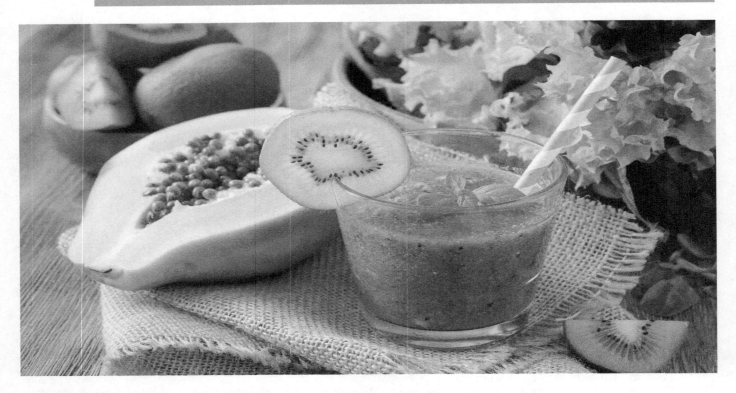

Preparation Time: 10 mins

Ingredients for 2 people:

- *250 g of ripe papaya*
- *1 ripe kiwi*
- *1 date*
- *2 handfuls (approx. 60 g) young spinach*
- *3 tbsp amaranth or quinoa flakes*
- *300 ml (1.5% fat) kefir*
- *1 tbsp hemp seeds*
- *2 tbsp raspberries*
- *1 tbsp coconut chips*

1. Halve the papaya and remove the seeds with a teaspoon. Peel the papaya, cut half of the pulp into pieces, put the rest aside for garnish.
2. Peel and slice the kiwi, set aside a few slices for garnish.
3. Core the date and cut it into small pieces (omit if you are fructose intolerant).
4. Sort the spinach, wash and pat dry, remove coarse stalks.
5. Finely puree the papaya, kiwi and date pieces, spinach leaves, amaranth or quinoa flakes and the kefir in a blender or in a tall mixing bowl with a hand blender.
6. Cut the remaining papaya into wedges. Lightly pound the hemp seeds in a mortar.
7. Divide the smoothie into two bowls and garnish with papaya wedges, kiwi slices and raspberries.
8. Serve sprinkled with hemp seeds and coconut chips.

Nutritional Value per Serving

380 Kcal	14 g Fat	34g Carbs	15g Protein	10g Fiber	3 BE

Millet Porridge with Fruit and Nuts

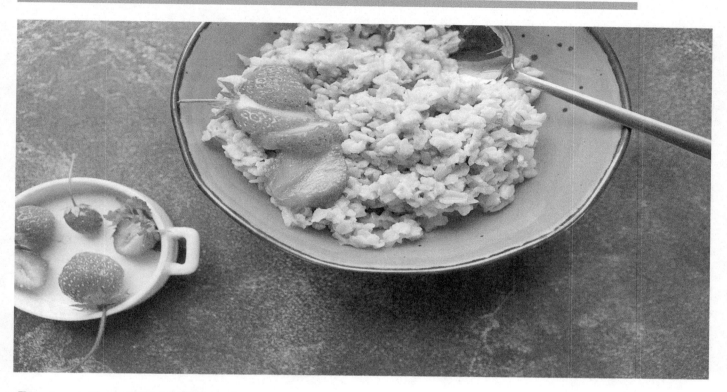

Preparation Time: 10 mins

Ingredients for 1 person:

- *60 g millet*
- *150 ml water*
- *20 g Flaked almonds*
- *150 g Berries, e.g., strawberries*
- *150 g (1.5% fat) natural yogurt*
- *1 pinch salt*
- *1 pinch cinnamon*
- *1 tsp DHA addition (omega-safe) linseed oil*

1. Rinse the millet hot in a sieve.
2. Bring to the boil with the water and a pinch of salt in a saucepan and simmer on medium heat for about 10 minutes. Let it swell briefly.
3. In the meantime, roast the flaked almonds in a pan without adding any fat. Let cool down.
4. Wash and clean the strawberries and cut them into small pieces. If necessary, puree other berries such as raspberries and pass them through a sieve to remove the stones.
5. Mix millet with yogurt and linseed oil and place in a bowl. Serve with the berries and flaked almonds.

Nutritional Value per Serving

497 Kcal	21 g Fat	57g Carbs	18g Protein	8 g Fiber

Immune Smoothie

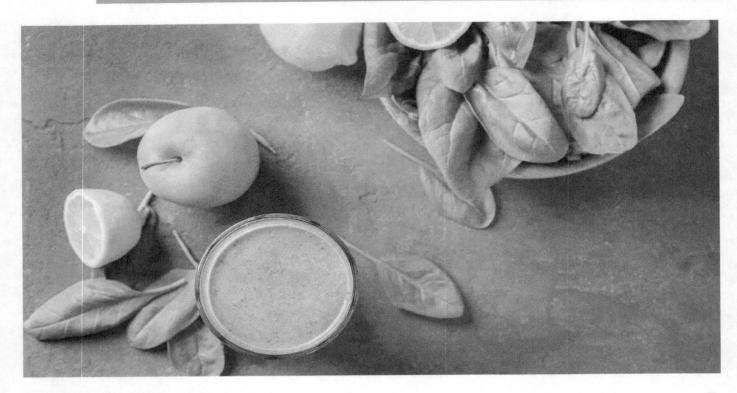

Preparation Time: 60 mins

Ingredients for 2 people:

- 1 apple
- ½ banana
- Juice of ½ lemon
- if you like: ginger
- 2 handfuls of spinach
- ½ teaspoon cinnamon
- water

1. Quarter and core the apple, peel the banana, wash the spinach and roughly chop.
2. Peel the ginger and cut it into small pieces.
3. Finely puree with lemon juice, water and cinnamon in a blender.

Nutritional Value

140 Kcal	0,3g Fat	31g Carbs	2g Protein	4g Fiber

Cottage Cheese Breakfast

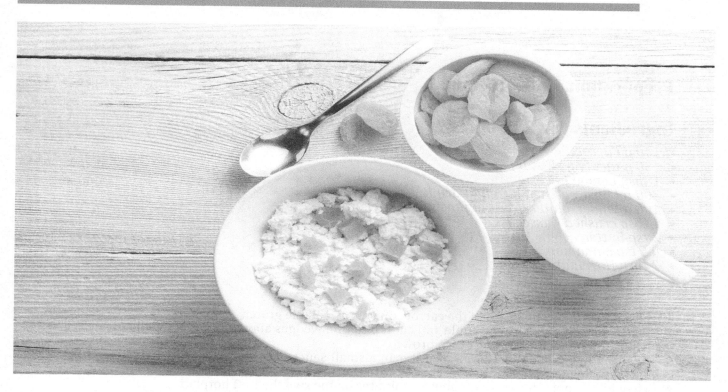

Preparation Time: 5 mins

Ingredients for 2 people

- *30 g Coconut chips*
- *60 g hearty oat flakes*
- *200 g grainy (semi-fat) cream cheese*
- *150 g (1.5% fat) natural yogurt*
- *200 g Apricots*
- *10 g ginger*
- *2 tsp Liquid honey*
- *0.5 tsp Cinnamon powder*
- *0.25 tsp Cardamom powder*

Note: *Instead of apricots, fruits such as persimmons, nectarine, peaches, currants, blackberries, gooseberries, cherries or melons, as well as carrots, also fit.*

1.   Roast the oatmeal in a small pan without fat, stirring over medium heat, for 3 to 4 minutes until fragrant. Then take it out and let it cool on a plate.
2.   In the meantime, mix the cottage cheese and yogurt in a bowl.
3.   Wash the fruit and cut it into bite-sized pieces.
4.   Mix in the cottage cheese mix together with the coconut chips. Distribute everything on bowls.
5.   Peel the ginger and grate finely.
6.   Drop the flake mixture over the cottage cheese mix and drizzle with 1 teaspoon of honey.
7.   Sprinkle with the grated ginger, cinnamon and cardamom, and serve the breakfast.

Nutritional Value per Serving

415 Kcal	17 g Fat	41g Carbs	21g Protein	7g Fiber

Carrot and Apple Porridge with Cinnamon

Preparation Time: 15 mins

Ingredients for 2 people:

- 140 g Carrots
- 150 g tart (e.g., Elstar) apple
- 1 tbsp Lemon juice
- 300 ml unsweetened hazelnut drink
- 100 g tender, gluten-free oat flakes
- 1 tbsp crushed flaxseed
- 2 tsp butter
- 0.5 tsp cinnamon
- 2 tbsp Hazelnuts

1. Clean, peel and roughly grate the carrots on your vegetable grater.
2. Wash, quarter and core the apple and cut it into thin wedges about 0.5 cm. Immediately drizzle with the lemon juice so that they don't turn brown.
3. Heat the nut drink and 125 ml of water in a small saucepan. Stir in oatmeal, carrots and flaxseed. Bring everything to a boil once, then simmer with the lid closed on mild heat for 10-15 minutes.
4. Then let the porridge swell for about 5 minutes on the switched-off hotplate.
5. Meanwhile, melt the butter in a small pan.
6. Add the apple wedges, season with half of the cinnamon and sauté over mild heat for 2-3 minutes while turning. Roughly chop the hazelnuts.
7. Divide the porridge into bowls to serve.
8. Place the apple wedges on top, sprinkle everything with the nuts and dust with the rest of the cinnamon.

Nutritional Value per Serving

460 Kcal	21 g Fat	50g Carbs	12g Protein	11 g Fiber

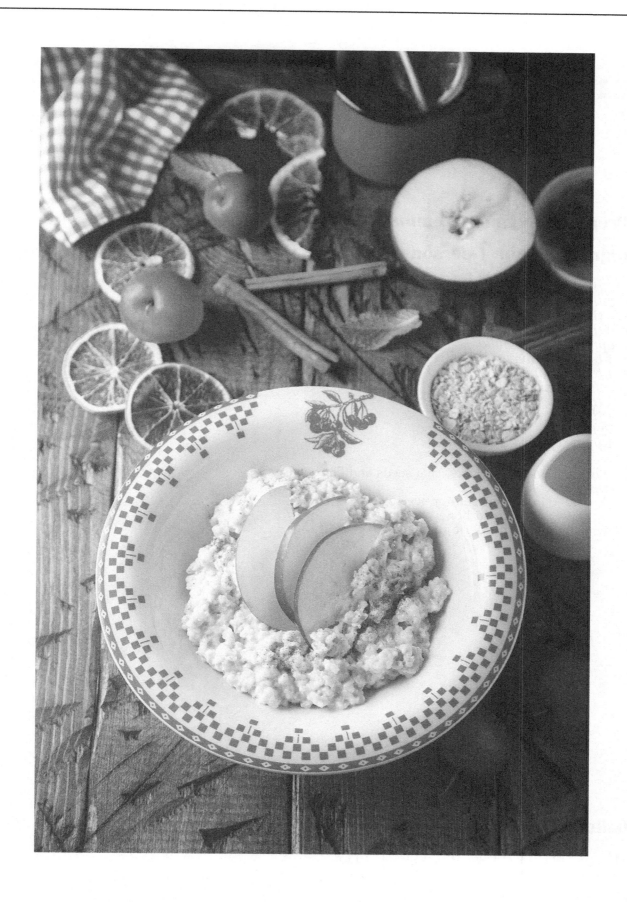

Cereal Porridge

Preparation Time: 10 mins

Ingredients for 1 person

- *2 tbsp oatmeal*
- *2 tbsp spelt flakes*
- *1 tbsp chia seeds*
- *2 tbsp flaxseed*
- *approx. 150 ml milk*
- *1 teaspoon honey*
- *1 teaspoon (slightly de-oiled, without sugar) cocoa powder*
- *1 tbsp linseed oil*
- *1 tbsp wheat germ oil*
- *½ teaspoon turmeric*
- *1 pinch of black pepper*

1. Soak oat and spelt flakes, chia seeds and flax seeds in the milk.
2. Let stand in the refrigerator overnight.
3. In the morning, add honey, cocoa powder, linseed oil, wheat germ oil, turmeric and pepper.

Nutritional Value

504 Kcal	39g Fat	44g Carbs	15g Protein	11 g Fiber

Crunchy Granola

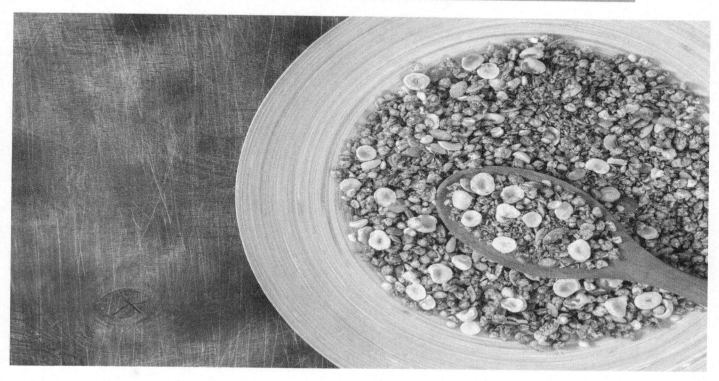

Preparation Time: 50 mins

Ingredients (for 5 servings, 1 serving = approx. 90 g):

- *1 banana*
- *3 tbsp coconut oil*
- *1 tbsp honey*
- *100 g of oatmeal*
- *3 tbsp flaxseed*
- *3 tbsp pumpkin seeds*
- *3 tbsp sunflower seeds*
- *3 tbsp puffed amaranth*
- *30 g of chopped almonds*
- *1 teaspoon cinnamon*

1. Preheat the oven to 150 degrees.
2. Peel the banana and mash it with coconut oil and honey.
3. Add all other ingredients and mix very well.
4. Spread on a parchment-lined baking sheet and bake in the oven for about 25 minutes. Stir every 10 minutes so that nothing burns - check in between.
5. When the muesli is browned, take it out of the oven and let it cool down well. When it cools down, it gets nice and crispy!
6. When it is completely cool, pour the muesli into an airtight container.

Tip : *There are many variations, for example, with sesame or other nuts.*

Nutritional Value per Servings

286 Kcal	15 g Fat	24g Carbs	10g Protein	5g Fiber

Fresh Pea Puree - Smarter with Cress and Lemon

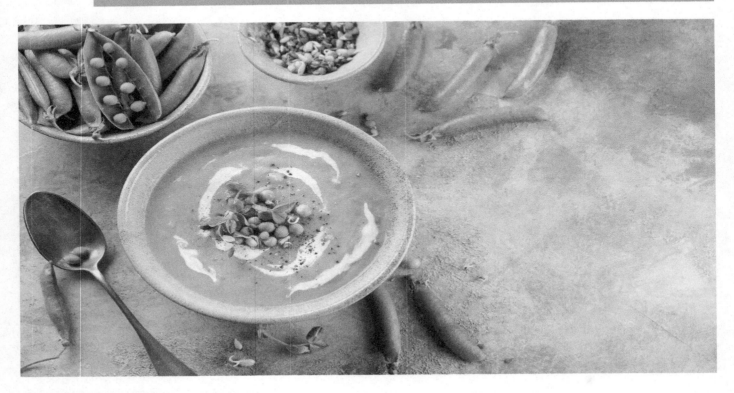

Preparation Time: 15 mins

Ingredients for 2 people

- *1 small clove of garlic*
- *1 small onion*
- *1 organic lemon*
- *1 tbsp*
- *olive oil*
- *250 g peas (frozen)*
- *4 tbsp soy cream*
- *Salt & pepper*
- *1 box garden cress*

1. Peel and finely chop the garlic and onion.
2. Wash the lemon, rub dry and finely grate the peel.
3. Halve the lemon and squeeze out 1 half (use the 2nd half for something else).
4. Heat oil in a pan. Sauté the garlic and onions in it over medium heat until translucent.
5. Add frozen peas and sauté for 1 minute.
6. Add 2 tablespoons of water, 1 tablespoon of lemon juice and the lemon zest and cook for 1–2 minutes.
7. Pour in the soy cream and briefly bring to a boil.
8. Put everything in a tall container and puree finely with a hand blender.
9. Season with salt and pepper.
10. Cut the cress from the bed with kitchen scissors, sprinkle over the pea puree and serve.

Nutritional Value per Serving

194 Kcal	9 g Fat	17g Carbs	9g Protein	7 g Fiber	0 g Added Sugar

Quinoa Curd Casserole with Fruit Salad

Preparation Time: 30 mins
Ready in 1h 10 min

Ingredients for 4 people:

- *150 g quinoa*
- *100 ml milk (1.5% fat)*
- *400 g oranges (2 oranges; 1 of them organic)*
- *2 eggs*
- *20 g brown cane sugar (1 tbsp)*
- *500 g low-fat quark*
- *½ tsp cinnamon*
- *½ tsp ground ginger*
- *liquid sweetener (at will)*
- *1 tsp germ oil*
- *2 tbsp raisins*
- *2 kiwi fruit*
- *200 g apples (1 apple)*
- *400 g bananas (2 bananas)*

1. Put the quinoa in a colander, rinse with hot water and drain.
2. Bring 200 ml of water and the milk to a boil in a saucepan and cook covered over low heat for 15 minutes.
3. Cover and leave to soak on the switched-off stove for another 5 minutes. Then let cool in the open pot.
4. While the quinoa is cooking, wash the organic orange with hot water, rub dry and finely rub about ¼ of the peel.
5. Separate the eggs and place the egg whites in a tall container. Beat with the whisk of the hand mixer until stiff, gradually pouring in the sugar.
6. Mix the quark and egg yolks with the quinoa. Season with grated orange peel, cinnamon and ginger. Fold in the whipped egg whites and add sweetener to taste.
7. Grease a flat casserole dish (approx. 1.5 l capacity) with the oil and pour in the quinoa quark mixture. Bake in a preheated oven at 200 ° C (convection 180 ° C, gas: level 3) for about 30 minutes.
8. In the meantime, peel both oranges so thick that all white is removed. Cut out the fruit fillets between the separating membranes and collect the juice in a bowl. Add the orange fillets. Roughly chop the raisins and also add to the bowl.
9. Peel and halve the kiwifruit and cut it into wedges. Wash the apple, rub dry, quarter, core and also cut into fine wedges. Fold both under the orange fillets.
10. Peel the bananas, cut them into slices, add to the bowl and let everything steep for about 10 minutes.
11. Serve the fruit salad with the quinoa quark casserole.

Nutritional Value

482 Kcal	7 g Fat	73g Carbs	27g Protein	7,5g Fiber	10 g Add Sugar

Salad Bowl with Watermelon and Grainy Cream Cheese

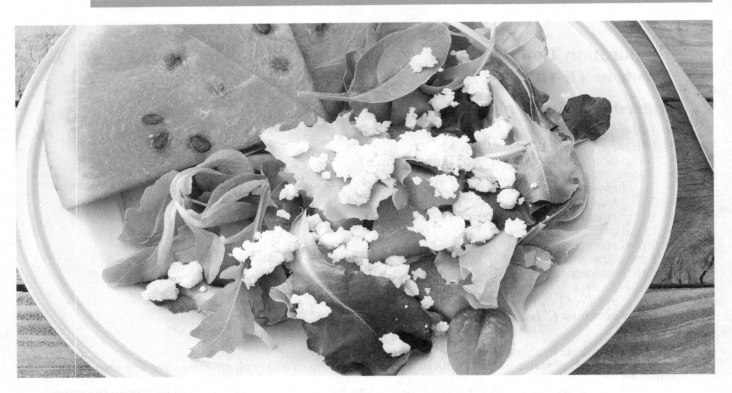

Preparation Time: 20 mins

Ingredients for 2 people:

- *100 g radish (1 piece)*
- *250 g mixed lettuce*
- *300 g watermelon (1 piece)*
- *150 g grainy cream cheese (13% fat)*
- *1 yellow pepper*
- *30 g ginger (1 piece)*
- *1 lime*
- *1 tbsp soy sauce*
- *1 tbsp Thai fish sauce*
- *Salt & pepper*
- *3 tbsp olive oil*
- *1 tsp sesame oil*
- *½ fret coriander*

1. Peel and clean the radish and cut it into fine slices.
2. Sprinkle with a bit of salt in a bowl and let steep for 10 minutes.
3. In the meantime, clean, wash and spin dry the salads.
4. Peel the watermelon and cut it into 1 cm cubes, removing the seeds.
5. Quarter the pepper, clean, core, wash and cut into fine strips or cubes.
6. For the vinaigrette, peel the ginger and grate it finely. Squeeze the lime. Mix the ginger, 2 tbsp lime juice, soy sauce, fish sauce, a little salt and pepper. Withhold both oils.
7. Drain the radish. Mix with the other ingredients and the vinaigrette in a bowl.
8. Wash the coriander, shake dry, pluck the leaves and spread over the salad with the cream cheese.

Nutritional Value per Serving

317 Kcal	21 g Fat	17g Carbs	14g Protein	7,5g Fiber	0g Added Sugar

Roasted Yeast Plaited Slices with Strawberries and Mint Quark

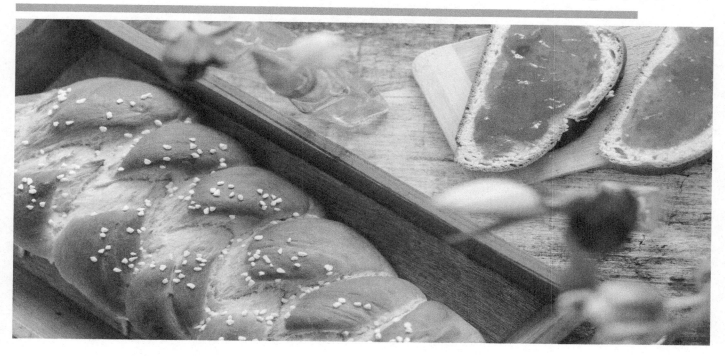

Preparation Time: 25 mins

Ingredients for 6 people:

- *750 g strawberries*
- *75 g pistachio nuts*
- *400 g hefezopf*
- *½ lemon*
- *300 g low-fat quark*
- *3 tbsp mint syrup*
- *2 stems mint*

1. Squeeze the lemon. Mix 2 tablespoons of juice with quark and mint syrup with a whisk until smooth.
2. Wash the mint, shake dry, pluck the leaves, chop finely and mix with the quark.
3. Wash, clean and halve the strawberries.
4. Roughly chop the pistachios.
5. Cut the yeast plait into slices and briefly roast vigorously on each side on the hot grill.
6. Brush each slice with quark, sprinkle strawberries on top and sprinkle with pistachios.

Nutritional Value per Serving

368 Kcal	13 g Fat	45g Carbs	14g Protein	5.5 g Fiber	8g Added Sugar

Pasta Dishes

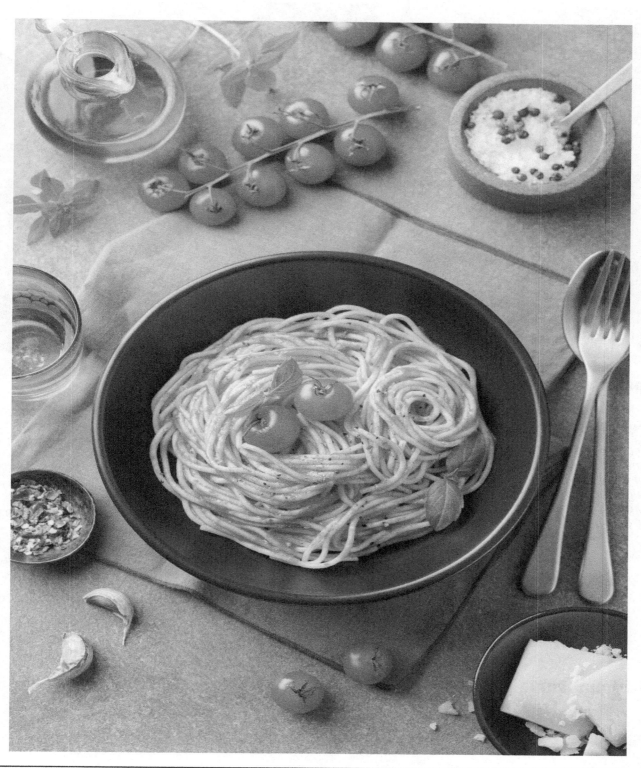

Sheep Cheese Pasta

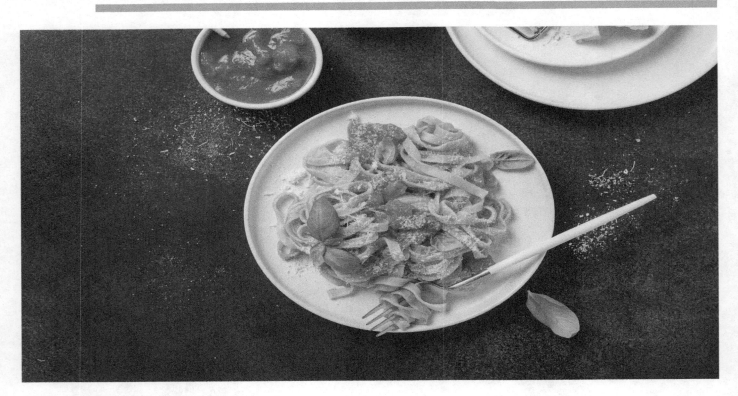

Preparation Time: 15 min

Ingredients per 2 people

- *150 g sun-dried tomatoes in oil*
- *2 small cloves of garlic*
- *15 g basil (1 bunch)*
- *120 g sheep cheese (45% fat in dry matter)*
- *200 g whole grain pasta (e.g., spaghetti)*
- *Salt & pepper*

1. Drain the tomatoes in a colander while collecting the oil in a small bowl.
2. Roughly chop the tomatoes with a sharp knife or cut them into strips.
3. Peel garlic and chop finely. Wash the basil, shake dry, pluck the leaves and roughly chop.
4. Crumble the sheep cheese with your fingers.
5. Cook the pasta in plenty of salted water according to the instructions on the packet until it is al dente.
6. In the meantime, measure 2 teaspoons of the collected tomato oil and heat in a pan over low heat.
7. Lightly sauté the garlic and tomatoes in it.
8. Add the basil and sheep cheese.
9. Drain the pasta, drain, mix in and season the sheep's cheese pasta with pepper.

Nutritional Value per Serving

595 Kcal	23 g Fat	70g Carbs	26g Protein	16 g Fiber	0g Added Sugar

Spaghetti with Swiss Chard in Mushroom and Cream Sauce

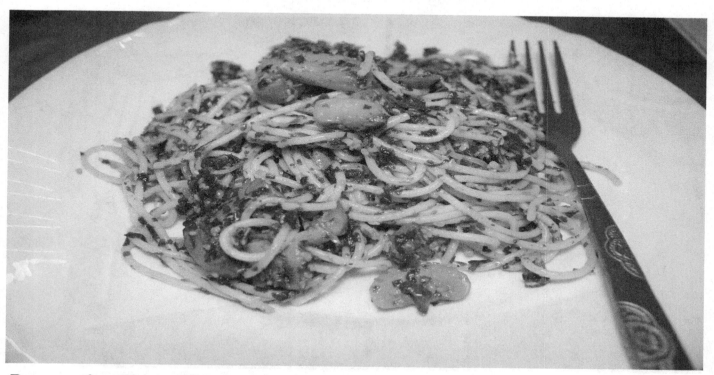

Preparation Time: 30 min
Ready in 35 min

Ingredients for 4 people:

- *300 g whole wheat spaghetti or whole wheat ribbon noodles*
- *100 g creme fraiche cheese*
- *1 shallot*
- *200 g shiitake mushrooms*
- *500 g swiss chard 1 small perennial*
- *Salt & pepper*
- *1 tbsp olive oil*
- *2 tsp mild curry powder*
- *50 ml vegetable broth*

1. Peel and finely dice the shallot.
2. Clean mushrooms. Cut off the stems, halve or quarter the hats depending on the size.
3. Wash the chard, remove the stems, cut the leaves into small pieces. Add plenty of salted water to the whole wheat pasta.
4. Heat the oil in a coated pan. Sauté shallot in it briefly over medium heat. Add mushrooms and fry. Dust the curry over it and fry it.
5. Stir in the chard leaves. Add the stock and crème fraîche and season everything with salt and pepper. Stew over medium heat for 8-10 minutes.
6. In the meantime, cook the whole wheat pasta in the boiling salted water according to the instructions on the packet.
7. Drain the pasta in a sieve, catch 2–3 tablespoons of pasta water and stir into the chard and mushroom sauce. D
8. rain the whole wheat pasta well and serve with the chard.

Nutritional Value per Serving

400 Kcal	11g Fat	55g Carbs	12g Protein	12 g Fiber	0g Added Sugar

Tuna Pasta in Spicy Tomato Sauce

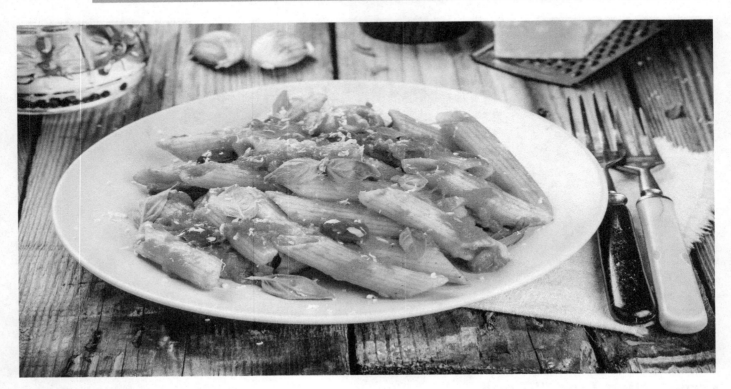

Preparation Time: 25 min

Ingredients per 2 person

- *200 g tuna in its own juice*
- *75 g green olives with stone*
- *175 g penne (preferably whole grain)*
- *20 g capers (glass)*
- *250 g tomatoes (3 tomatoes)*
- *100 ml tomato juice*
- *Salt & pepper*
- *1 onion*
- *½ fret basil*
- *2 tbsp olive oil*

1. Drain the tuna well.
2. Cut the olives into slices from the stone.
3. Cook the pasta in plenty of salted water according to the instructions on the packet until al dente.
4. While the pasta is cooking, peel and finely dice the onion. Wash and quarter the tomatoes, removing the stalks. Core and roughly dice tomatoes.
5. Wash the basil, shake dry, pluck the leaves and chop finely.
6. Heat the oil in a pan over medium heat. Sauté onion cubes in it for 1 minute until colorless. Add diced tomatoes and cook for 1 minute more.
7. Add olives, capers and tomato juice and simmer over low heat for 5 minutes.
8. Add the tuna and simmer until the tuna is completely warmed up.
9. Drain the pasta in a sieve, drain well and mix with the tomato sauce.
10. Season with salt and pepper and serve sprinkled with basil.

Nutritional Value per Serving

622 Kcal	28 g Fat	59g Carbs	30g Protein	13g Fiber	0g Added Sugar

Pasta and Vegetable Salad with Fried Red Mullet Fillets

Preparation Time: 35 min
Ready in 45 min

Ingredients for 2 people:

- *100 g whole wheat pasta*
- *200 g red mullet fillet (4 red mullet fillets)*
- *200 g small cucumber (about half cucumber)*
- *1 yellow pepper*
- *175 g cherry tomatoes*
- *2 spring onions*
- *1 small clove of garlic*
- *2 stems basil*
- *50 ml tomato juice*
- *4 tbsp olive oil*
- *1 tbsp red wine vinegar*
- *Salt & pepper*

1. Preparation steps
2. Cook the pasta in plenty of boiling salted water according to the instructions on the package, drain it in a sieve and let it drain.
3. In the meantime, wash the cucumber and cut it in half. Peel one half, cut lengthways and remove the kernels with a tablespoon. Cut the cucumber into small cubes.
4. Quarter, core, wash and cut the pepper into small cubes.
5. Wash the cherry tomatoes and cut them in half.
6. Clean and wash the spring onions and cut the white and light green into thin slices. Mix the cucumber, bell pepper, tomatoes and spring onions with the noodles in a bowl.
7. Peel and finely chop the clove of garlic. Wash the basil, shake dry, pluck the leaves off and roughly chop.
8. Whisk the garlic and basil with the tomato juice, 3 tablespoons of oil, vinegar, salt and pepper.
9. Mix the salad dressing with the vegetables and pasta and let it steep for 15 minutes (marinate).
10. Heat the rest of the olive oil in a pan and season the red mullet fillets with salt and pepper.
11. Fry the fish fillets in the hot oil for 2 minutes on each side. Remove and serve with the salad.

Nutritional Value per Serving

467 Kcal	20 g Fat	39g Carbs	30g Protein	10.5g Fiber	0g Added Sugar

Tagliatelle with Radicchio in Creamy Ham Sauce

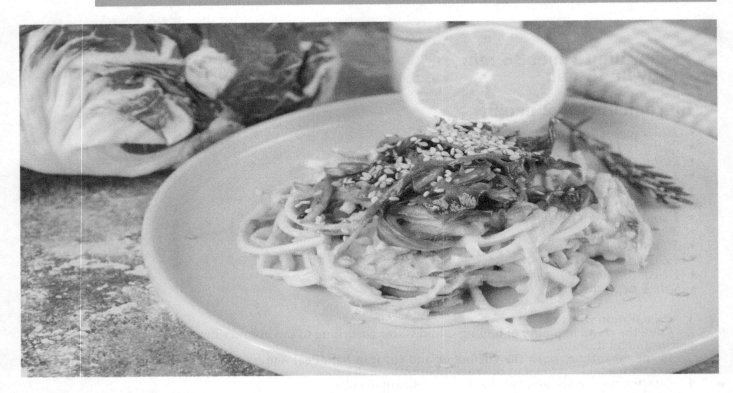

Preparation Time: 25 mins

Ingredients for 2 people:

- 1 small head radicchio
- 2 small red onions
- 1 tbsp pine nuts
- 75 g salmon ham (without fat rim)
- 175 g pappardelle
- Salt & pepper
- 2 tbsp olive oil
- 100 ml dry white wine or grape juice
- 150 ml soy cream
- ½ lemon

1. Wash the radicchio, cut in half and remove the stalk. Cut the radicchio crosswise into fine strips.
2. Peel the onions and cut them into fine strips. Roast the pine nuts in a dry pan until golden, leave to cool on a plate.
3. Cut the salmon ham into 1 cm wide strips. Cook the pasta in plenty of salted water according to the instructions on the packet.
4. In the meantime, heat the oil in a pan and sauté the onion strips over medium heat for 4 minutes until they are colorless. Add radicchio and sauté for 1 minute.
5. Pour white wine into the pan and let it boil down completely in 5-10 minutes.
6. Add soy cream to the pan and cook for 2 minutes.
7. Add the ham and cook for 1 minute more. Squeeze the lemon. Season the sauce with salt, pepper and 2 teaspoons of lemon juice.
8. Drain the pasta in a sieve and mix with the sauce. Serve sprinkled with pine nuts.

Nutritional Value per Serving

634 Kcal	31 g Fat	64g Carbs	21g Protein	11 g Fiber	0g Added Sugar

Main Courses

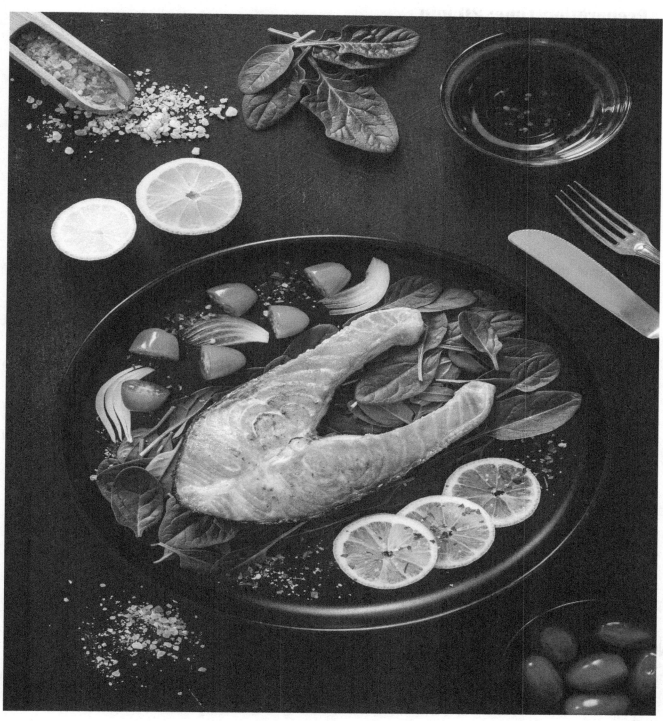

Eggplant Casserole with Mozzarella

Preparation Time: 20 min

Ingredients for 4 people:

- *750 g eggplant*
- *1 onion*
- *1 toe garlic*
- *3 tbsp olive oil*
- *400 g (canned) tomatoes*
- *200 g Mozzarella*
- *20 g freshly grated parmesan*
- *salt*
- *freshly ground pepper*
- *dried oregano*
- *fresh basil*

1. Preheat the oven to 220 degrees circulating air or 200 degrees (top / bottom heat). Wash the aubergines, pat dry, clean and cut into finger-thick slices.
2. Place on a baking sheet lined with baking paper and grill in the oven for 5-7 minutes on both sides. When they turn color, the eggplants are done. Do not turn off the stove.
3. In the meantime, peel the onion and garlic, cut the onion into rings and finely dice the garlic (omit onions and garlic if you have gastritis).
4. Wash the basil and shake dry, pluck the leaves and cut into fine strips.
5. Carefully heat the oil in a pan and sauté the onion rings and garlic. Add the peeled tomatoes, season everything with salt, pepper, oregano and basil and simmer uncovered over low heat for 8-10 minutes.
6. Cut the mozzarella into thin slices (if you have reflux / heartburn, use reduced-fat mozzarella).
7. Brush a casserole dish thinly with oil, add 2 tablespoons of tomato sauce, cover with a layer of aubergine slices. Layer 2-3 tablespoons of tomato sauce, mozzarella slices and 2 tablespoons of grated parmesan on top. Continue doing this until all the food has been consumed. The top layer is made up of mozzarella and parmesan.
8. Bake in the preheated oven (center) for 15-20 minutes.

Nutritional Value per Serving

290 Kcal	20 g Fat	8g Carbs	16g Protein	4 g Fiber

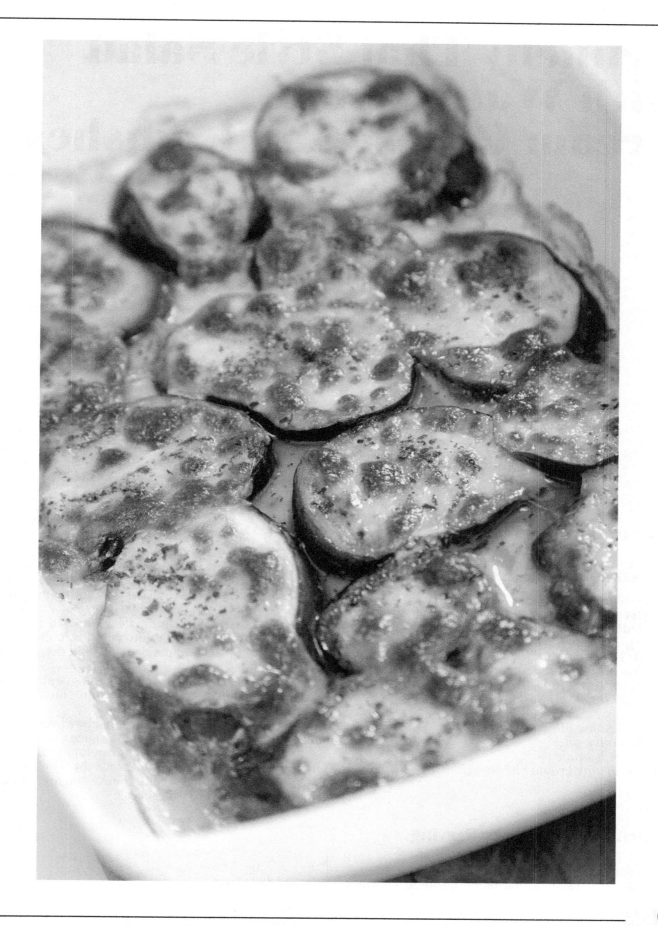

Crunchy Thai-Style Salad with Watermelon, Cream Cheese and Radishes

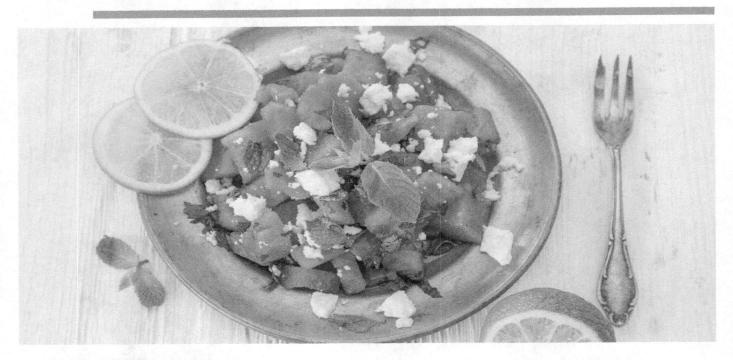

Preparation Time: 30 mins

Ingredients for 2 people:

- 1 bunch radish
- 1 piece watermelon (approx. 200 g pulp)
- 1 small red onion
- 150 g arugula
- ½ fret flat-leaf parsley
- 2 tbsp black sesame
- 1-piece fresh ginger (approx. 2 cm long)
- 1 small lime
- 1 ½ tbsp soy sauce
- 1 tsp sesame oil
- 2 tbsp olive oil
- 1 tsp chili sauce
- 150 g grainy cream cheese (13% fat)

1. Wash and clean the radishes and cut them into fine slices.
2. Core the melon and cut the flesh into balls.
3. Peel the onion and cut it into very fine cubes.
4. Wash the rocket and parsley and spin dry. Pluck the parsley leaves.
5. Roast the sesame seeds in a pan, remove and let cool.
6. Peel the ginger, grate it finely and squeeze it out vigorously by hand. Squeeze the lime.
7. Mix the ginger and lime juice in a bowl with the soy sauce, sesame oil, olive oil and chili sauce.
8. Mix the rocket, parsley, watermelon, radishes and onion cubes with the sauce and place them on a plate.
9. Spread the grainy cream cheese on top, sprinkle with the sesame seeds and serve.

Nutritional Value per Serving

372 Kcal	23 g Fat	22g Carbs	16g Protein	6.5 g Fiber	0g Added Sugar

Salmon Steak with Swiss Chard Butter

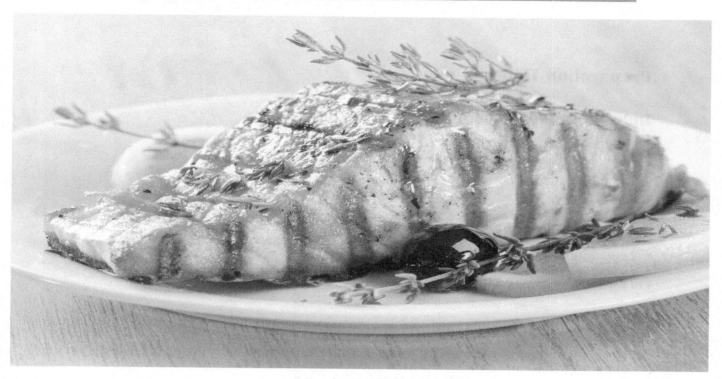

Preparation Time: 5 min

Ingredients for 4 people

- ½ lemon
- 4 (200 g each, with skin) salmon steaks
- 2 tbsp coconut oil

1. Squeeze the lemon half. Rinse the salmon steaks with cold water, pat dry, marinate with the lemon juice and refrigerate for about two hours.
2. Heat up the grill. Brush the salmon steaks with oil and fry briefly on each side over high heat on the grill.
3. Then place in a fire-proof dish (avoid using aluminum foil if possible) and let it stand for about 5 minutes.

1. **Tip:** *You can also prepare the salmon steaks in the house: simply fry them in the pan and let them steep in the oven.*

Preparation Time: 15 min

Ingredients for the chard butter:

- 4 small leaves of Swiss chard
- 125 g soft butter
- 2 teaspoons Worcester sauce
- ½ teaspoon salt
- ½ teaspoon white pepper
- 4 pinches of nutmeg

Nutritional Value

1. Wash, dry and chop the chard leaves. Mix with butter, Worcester sauce, salt, pepper and nutmeg.
2. Let the mixture cool in the refrigerator for 15 minutes.
3. Then shape the chard butter into a 15 cm long roll, wrap it in cling film and let it set in the freezer for about 3 hours.
4. Take out of the cooling compartment and remove the foil.
5. Cut 8-12 finger-thick slices from the roll, place on the grilled salmon steaks and serve

644 Kcal	53g Fat	2g Carbs	41g Protein

Rocket and Radicchio Salad with Grapefruit and Scallops

Preparation Time: 40 mins

Ingredients for 2 people:

- 8 scallops (without mussel shell)
- 4 grapefruit
- 1 tbsp granular dijon mustard
- 1 tbsp balsamic vinegar
- Salt & pepper
- 60 ml olive oil
- 1 handful arugula
- 1 radicchio
- 1 red onion
- 1 clove of garlic
- 1 tsp rapeseed oil

1. Squeeze the juice from 2 grapefruits. In a small saucepan, reduce the juice until it is syrupy over medium heat.
2. Mix grapefruit juice with mustard, vinegar, a little salt, pepper and olive oil to make a salad sauce (vinaigrette), set aside.
3. Clean the rocket, cutting off the lower ends of the stems.
4. Clean the radicchio, remove the outer leaves and cut out the stalk in a wedge shape. Wash salads, spin dry.
5. Cut the radicchio into fine strips. Put salads in a bowl.
6. Peel the rest of the grapefruit with a knife so that all of the white skin is removed. Cut the pulp into slices and roughly chop.
7. Peel the onion and slice it into very thin slices. Flatten the unpeeled clove of garlic with a knife.
8. Heat a coated pan and brush with rapeseed oil.
9. Pat the scallops dry and fry them in the hot pan with the garlic for 2 minutes on each side. Season with salt and pepper.
10. In the meantime, mix the salads and grapefruit pieces with the salad sauce.
11. Divide the salad among plates and place the mussels and onion slices on top.

Nutritional Value per Serving

515 Kcal	33g Fat	30g Carbs	16g Protein	3g Fiber	0g Added Sugar

Green Beans au Gratin on Spelt Semolina

Preparation Time: 15 min

Ingredients for 2 people:

- *300 g green beans (frozen)*
- *400 ml classic vegetable broth*
- *1 tsp dried thyme*
- *100 g wholemeal spelt semolina*
- *60 g blue cheese (50% fat)*
- *Salt & pepper*

1. Bring plenty of water to a boil in a saucepan, season with salt and add the beans.
2. Cook covered over medium heat for 8 minutes.
3. In the meantime, bring the vegetable stock with the thyme to a boil. Scatter spelt semolina while stirring and bring to a boil.
4. Cover and leave to swell over low heat for about 8 minutes, stirring occasionally.
5. In the meantime, cut the blue cheese into small cubes. Drain the beans in a colander.
6. Season spelt semolina with salt and pepper and place in a flat baking dish.
7. Spread the beans as wide strips on the semolina and pour the blue cheese over them.
8. Gratinate on the middle shelf under the preheated oven grill for 2-3 minutes until the cheese melts.
9. Take out and sprinkle with pepper

Nutritional Value

317 Kcal	11 g Fat	37g Carbs	16g Protein	9.5g Fiber	0g Added Sugar

Vegetable Sushi with Nori Seaweed

Preparation Time: 1 h
Ready in 1h 45 min

Ingredients for 2 people:

- *125 g sushi rice*
- *2 ½ tbsp rice vinegar*
- *1 tsp honey*
- *1 mini cucumber approx. 250 g*
- *1 small ripe avocado approx. 150 g*
- *6 sheets chicory*
- *1 small red pepper approx. 150 g*
- *75 g cream cheese (13% fat)*
- *2 tsp wasabi paste*
- *2 sheets nori seaweed*
- *½ tsp salt*
- *soy sauce*

1. Rinse the sushi rice in a colander with cold water until the water runs off. Drain in a sieve for about 20 minutes, then bring to a boil with 250 ml of water in a saucepan.
2. Cook for 2 minutes in an open saucepan, then cover and let soak for 20 minutes on the switched-off hotplate.
3. Take the pot off the stove, remove the lid and put a kitchen towel over it instead. Let stand for 10 minutes.
4. In a small saucepan, heat 2 tablespoons of rice vinegar, honey and salt until just before boiling, stirring until the honey and salt have dissolved.
5. Put the rice in a bowl and spread it apart so that it cools down faster. Pour the vinegar mixture over it and let it cool down to room temperature for about 30 minutes.
6. In the meantime, wash the cucumber thoroughly, rub dry and cut in half lengthways. Remove the seeds with a spoon and cut the pulp lengthways into thin strips with a peeler.
7. Halve the avocado and remove the stone, cut the pulp into slices. Immediately drizzle with the remaining rice vinegar to prevent discoloration.
8. Wash the chicory leaves, shake dry and cut into long strips about 0.5 cm wide.
9. Halve, core, wash and cut the pepper into long thin strips.
10. In a small bowl, stir the cream cheese with the wasabi paste until smooth.
11. Place 1 nori sheet on the bamboo mat and cover with half of the rice, leaving a small edge free at the top and bottom.
12. Spread half of the cream cheese mixture across the bottom third of the rice.
13. Spread the cucumber, avocado, chicory and bell pepper on top as well.
14. Shape everything into a thick roll with the help of the mat. Make a second roll from the remaining ingredients.
15. Dip a sharp knife in water and use it to cut the rolls into 8 equal pieces.
16. Serve with soy sauce.

Nutritional Value per Serving

264 Kcal	9 g Fat	36g Carbs	6g Protein	3.5g Fiber	3g Added Sugar

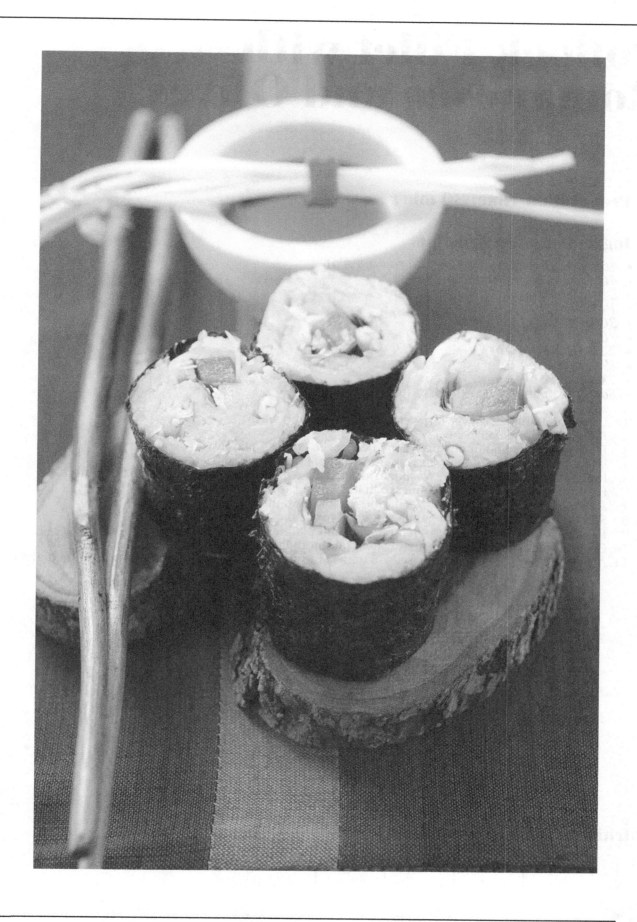

Pollock Fillet with Romanesco and Olives

Preparation Time: 30 min

Ingredients for 2 peolpe

- 400 g small romanesco (1 small romanesco)
- 40 g green olives (without stones)
- 2 small onions
- 1 clove of garlic
- 300 g pollock fillet
- 20 g almond kernels
- 2 stems marjoram
- ½ lemon
- 2 tbsp olive oil
- Salt & pepper

1. Clean the Romanesco, cut into very small florets and wash.
2. Roughly chop the olives.
3. Peel the onions and finely dice them. Peel garlic and chop finely.
4. Wash the fish fillet, pat dry and cut into 3 cm pieces.
5. Roughly chop the almonds. Wash marjoram, shake dry, pluck leaves. Squeeze the lemon.
6. Heat oil in a pan. Fry the Romanesco in it, swirling, for 3–4 minutes over high heat.
7. Add the almonds, onions and garlic and fry for 1 minute. Season with salt and pepper.
8. Season the fish pieces with pepper and add to the pan with the olives.
9. Deglaze with 2 tablespoons of lemon juice and 2 tablespoons of water.
10. Cover immediately and cook on low heat for another 4–5 minutes.
11. At the end of the cooking time, season with salt, sprinkle with marjoram and serve immediately.

Nutritional Value per Serving

373 Kcal	20 g Fat	7g Carbs	39g Protein	8g Fiber	0g Added Sugar

Salmon on Fennel and Carrot Vegetables

Preparation Time: 20 mins

Ingredients for 2 people:

- *300 g salmon fillet*
- *3 medium-sized carrots*
- *½ bulb of fennel*
- *1 small onion*
- *1 clove of garlic*
- *1 tbsp rapeseed oil*
- *1 tbsp olive oil*
- *Salt & pepper*
- *1 tbsp sour cream*
- *1 teaspoon chopped dill*
- *Preheat the oven to 180 degrees.*

1. Wash and clean the carrots and fennel and cut into very thin slices. Peel the onion and cut into fine strips, mash the garlic.
2. Divide the salmon into two equal steaks, season with salt and pepper and about 10 to 12 minutes without fat in oven and cook until it browns slightly (alternatively, you can him in a heated pan with a little oil until light brown.)
3. While the salmon cooked, sauté the vegetables in a little water and the oil for about 10 minutes until al dente. Add sour cream and dill and season with salt and pepper.
4. Arrange the salmon fillets on the carrot and fennel vegetables. Jacket potatoes go well with it. If you have gastritis, choose rice as a side dish instead.

Nutritional Value per Serving

428 Kcal	29 g Fat	11g Carbs	32g Protein	5g Fiber

Oat Pancakes With Herb Quark

Preparation Time: 30 min

Ingredients for 2 people

- 50 g fine oatmeal
- 50 g hearty oat flakes
- 150 ml Vegetable broth
- 20 g Oat bran
- 1 Spring onion
- 2 tbsp olive oil
- 1 egg
- 2 tbsp Sunflower seeds
- 1 tbsp finely chopped parsley
- Salt & pepper
- noble sweet paprika powder

1. Mix the oat flakes, pour the boiling vegetable stock over them and cover and leave to soak for 30 minutes. Drain and drain. Stir in the oat bran.
2. Wash and clean the spring onions, finely chop the white and cut the green into fine rings. Sauté briefly in 1 teaspoon of oil until the green is soft and add to the oatmeal mixture. Mix in the egg, sunflower seeds and herbs well and season with salt, pepper and a little paprika powder.
3. Shape the mixture into 2 patties and fry them in the remaining oil on each side for about 5 minutes until golden brown.

Nutritional Value per Serving:

434 Kcal	22 g Fat	42g Carbs	16g Protein	9 g Fiber

Preparation Time: 10 min

Ingredients for the quark:

- 300 g low-fat quark
- 1 Tbsp low-fat (1.5% fat) milk
- 1 bunch chives
- Salt & pepper
- 2 tsp Linseed or walnut oil

1. Mix the quark with the milk and oil until smooth. Wash the chives, pat dry and cut into fine rolls. Mix with the quark and season with salt and pepper.
2. Alternatively, 1 to 2 tablespoons of Italian herbs (frozen food) can be used instead of chives.

Nutritional Value per Serving

170 Kcal	6 g Fat	6g Carbs	22g Protein	0.6g Fiber	0.5 BE

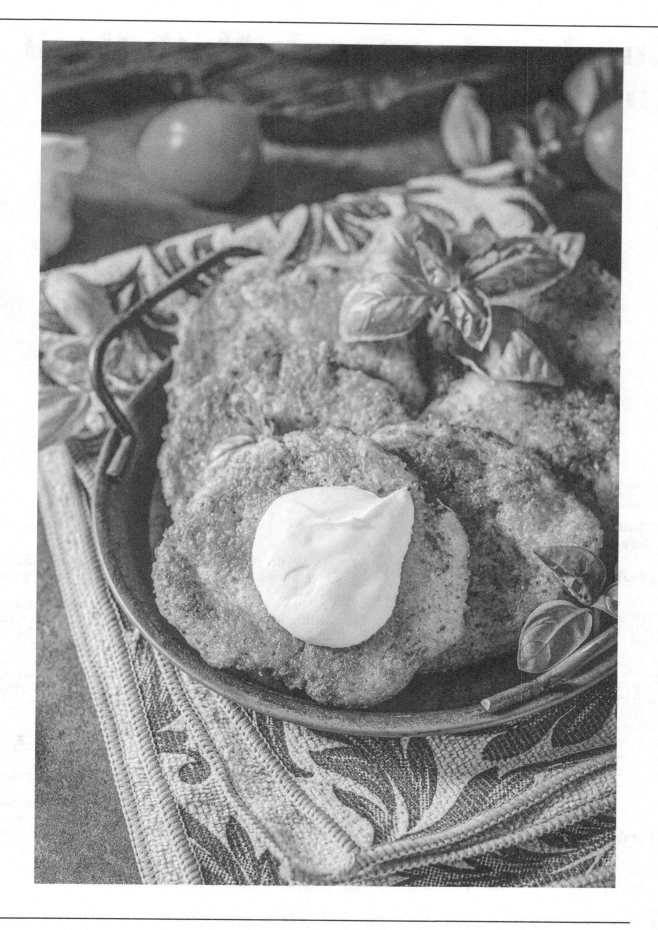

Zucchini Carpaccio With Basil And Ricotta Dumplings

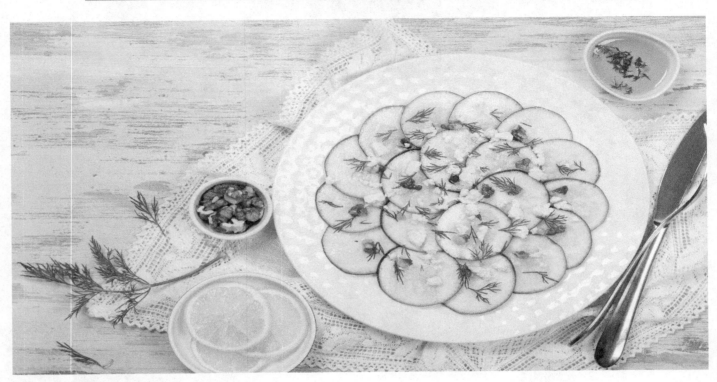

Preparation Time: 25 min
Ready in 35 min

Ingredients for 4 people:

- 300 g small green courgettes (2 small green courgettes)
- 150 g yellow small zucchini (1 small yellow zucchini)
- 3 tbsp olive oil
- Salt & pepper
- 30 g pickled sun-dried tomatoes
- 30 g green olives (without stones)
- ½ fret basil
- 175 g ricotta
- 1 dried chili pepper
- 20 g pine nuts
- 20 g rocket

1. Wash the zucchini and cut off the ends. Cut lengthways into 5 mm thin slices with the vegetable slicer.
2. Place the zucchini slices on a baking sheet, brush with a little oil and season with salt and pepper. Bake in the preheated oven at 220 ° C (fan oven 200 ° C, gas: level 3–4) on the middle shelf for 8 minutes. Take out and let cool.
3. Drain the sun-dried tomatoes. Finely chop the olives.
4. Wash the basil, shake dry, pluck the leaves off and chop finely.
5. Chop the drained tomatoes very finely.
6. Mix tomatoes, olives and basil with ricotta in a bowl, season with salt, pepper and some crumbled chili pepper.
7. Roast pine nuts in a pan without fat. Clean, wash and spin dry the rocket.
8. Place the zucchini slices on a plate. Using 2 moistened tablespoons, cut off the dumplings from the ricotta mixture and place them on the plates with the zucchini.
9. Garnish with pine nuts and rocket.

Nutritional Value per Serving

196 Kcal	15 g Fat	6g Carbs	9g Protein	3 g Fiber	0g Added Sugar

Monkfish Schnitzel with Yellow Tomatoes

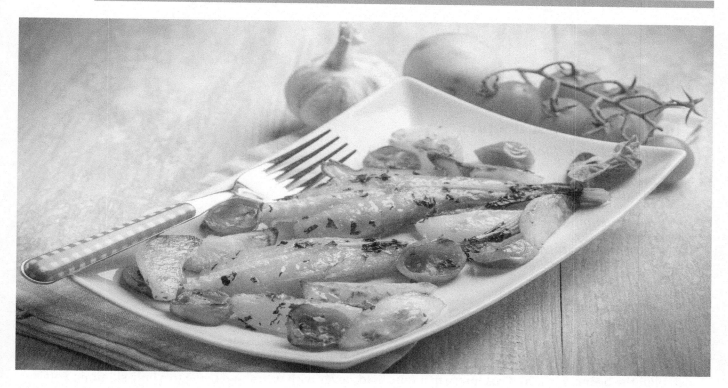

Preparation Time: 35 min

Ingredients for 2 people:

- *275 g monkfish fillet*
- *14 yellow cherry tomatoes*
- *25 g capers (glass)*
- *125 ml white wine or fish stock*
- *1 shallot*
- *4 stems parsley*
- *½ lemon*
- *½ orange*
- *1 tsp coriander seeds*
- *5 black peppercorns*
- *2 tbsp olive oil*
- *Salt & pepper*

1. Wash the tomatoes, cut them in half and squeeze out the seeds.
2. Drain the capers and roughly chop them.
3. Peel the shallot and chop it very finely. Wash parsley, shake dry, pluck leaves and roughly chop. Squeeze the lemon and orange separately.
4. Wash the monkfish, pat dry and cut into 2 cm thick slices. Cover the slices with cling film and flatten it a little with a meat tenderizer or cake server. Coarsely crush the coriander seeds and peppercorns in a mortar.
5. Turn the fish slices in the spices.
6. Heat the oil in a non-stick pan and fry the fish slices on each side over high heat for 1 minute. Remove. Season to taste with a little salt and lemon juice.
7. Add tomatoes and shallot to the pan and cook for 30 seconds while stirring.
8. Stir 50 ml orange juice and white wine into the pan.
9. Add capers, bring to a boil and cook over high heat for 3 minutes. Put the fish and parsley in the pan and heat briefly. Season with salt and pepper and serve immediately.

Nutritional Value per Serving

240 Kcal	12 g Fat	6g Carbs	22g Protein	1.5 g Fiber	0g Added Sugar

Italian Bean And Tuna Salad With Celery And Tomatoes

Preparation Time: 1h

Ingredients for 2 people:

- *80 g dried cannellini beans*
- *1 clove of garlic*
- *1 branch rosemary*
- *2 tomatoes*
- *150 g celery (2 sticks)*
- *1 mini cucumber*
- *½ fret parsley*
- *1 tsp dijon mustard*
- *1 tbsp white wine vinegar*
- *Salt & pepper*
- *cane sugar*
- *3 tbsp olive oil*
- *160 g tuna in its own juice*

1. Put the beans in a bowl and soak in plenty of cold water overnight.
2. Drain the water the following day. Peel the garlic. Wash rosemary.
3. Put the beans, garlic and rosemary in a saucepan, cover with water and bring to a boil, skimming off the resulting foam with a slotted ladle if necessary.
4. Cook the beans over low heat for about 50 minutes so that they are cooked but still have a bit of bite.
5. In the meantime, wash the tomatoes and cut out the green stalks in a wedge shape. Quarter and core the tomatoes and cut them into pieces.
6. Wash, clean, remove the threads from the celery and slice or cut into very thin slices.
7. Wash, dry or peel the cucumber. Quarter and core the cucumber. Then cut the cucumber into fine cubes. Wash the parsley, shake dry and roughly chop the leaves.
8. Mix the mustard, vinegar, salt, pepper and sugar in a bowl. Withhold the olive oil.
9. Mix the salad sauce with the tomato pieces, cucumber cubes, celery slices and parsley.
10. Put the tuna in a colander and drain. Tear apart the tuna with a fork.
11. Drain the beans, remove the garlic and rosemary. Drain the beans well and let them cool for about 5 minutes, then mix with the other salad ingredients.
12. Season the salad with salt and pepper.
13. Finally, add the tuna to the salad and serve lukewarm.

Nutritional Value

400 Kcal	21 g Fat	22g Carbs	29g Protein	9.5g Fiber	2g Added Sugar

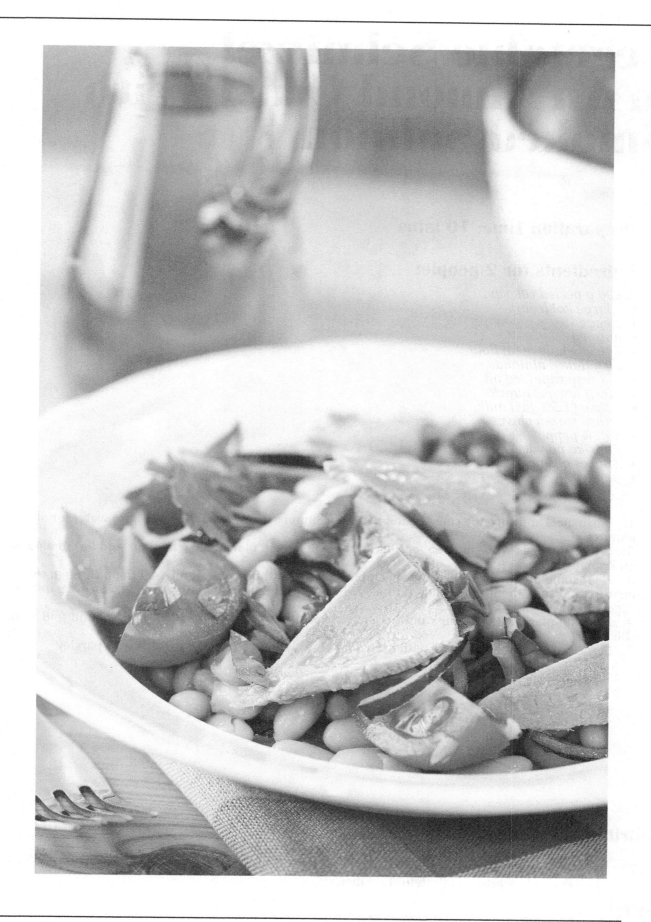

Vegetable Schnitzel in An Almond Crust With Smoked Salmon

Preparation Time: 10 mins

Ingredients for 2 people:

- *200 g peeled celeriac*
- *1 large kohlrabi*
- *2 eggs*
- *nutmeg*
- *2 tbsp whole meal flour*
- *80 g flaked almonds*
- *2-3 tbsp rapeseed oil*
- *300 g low-fat quark*
- *3 tbsp (1.5% fat) milk*
- *1 tbsp frozen chives*
- *Salt & pepper*
- *Paprika powder*
- *4 slices of smoked salmon*
- *parsley*

1. Wash, peel and slice the celeriac and kohlrabi. Simmer in a saucepan with a little water for about 5 minutes.
2. Whisk the eggs with salt, pepper and nutmeg on a deep plate. Place the flour and flaked almonds on 2 small plates.
3. Heat some oil in a pan. Dust the vegetable slices very thinly with flour, pull them through the egg mixture and turn them in the almond flakes. Pour into the hot pan and fry slowly, turning, until the vegetables are soft.
4. Mix the quark with the milk until creamy. Season with salt, pepper and paprika and fold in the chives.
5. Serve the vegetable schnitzel with herb quark and salmon slices and garnish with parsley.

Nutritional Value per 524g portion

720 Kcal	46g Fat	20g Carbs	51g Protein	12 g Fiber

Watercress and Cucumber Salad with Smoked Salmon

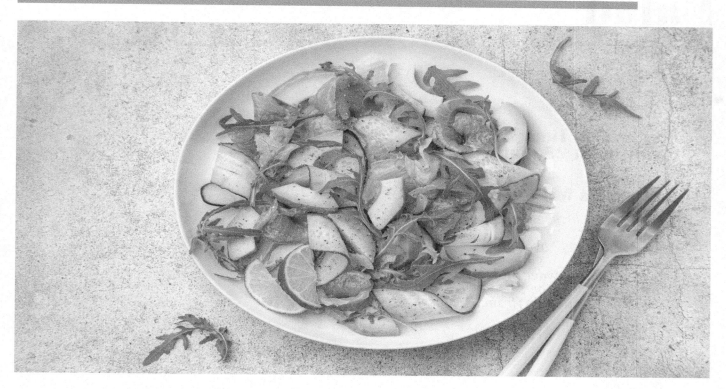

Preparation Time: 25 min

Ingredients for 2 people:

- 400 g cucumber (1 cucumber)
- 200 g watercress (2 bunch)
- 200 g sorrel (1 bunch)
- 1 small red onion
- 1 tbsp estragon mustard
- 2 tbsp white wine vinegar
- Salt & pepper
- 5 tbsp rapeseed oil
- 125 g smoked salmon (sliced)

1. Wash the cucumber thoroughly and cut it in half lengthways. Cut the cucumber into thin slices, lightly salt and drain in a colander for 15 minutes.
2. In the meantime, wash, clean and spin dry the watercress and sorrel. Cut into bite-sized pieces.
3. Peel and halve the onion and cut it into fine slices.
4. Mix together tarragon mustard, vinegar, salt and pepper.
5. Withhold the oil. Arrange the cucumber, watercress, sorrel, onion and smoked salmon decoratively on a platter.
6. Spread the vinaigrette on top and serve the salad immediately.

Nutritional Value per Serving

355 Kcal	30g Fat	5g Carbs	15g Protein	3.5g Fiber	0g Added Sugar

Tamarind Chicken Skewers With Avocado And Tomato Salad

Preparation Time: 45 min
Ready in 2h 25 min

Ingredients for 4 people:

- *400 g small chicken breast fillet (4 small chicken breast fillets)*
- *400 g avocado (2 avocados)*
- *2 limes*
- *2 tsp paprika powder (noble sweet)*
- *some cayenne peppers*
- *2 tbsp tamarind pulp (from the glass)*
- *5 tbsp ketchup*
- *275 g tomatoes (4 tomatoes)*
- *125 g red onion*
- *1 red pepper*
- *½ fret coriander*
- *Salt & pepper*

1. Put the wooden skewers in water. Wash the chicken breast fillets, pat dry, and cut into 2 cm cubes.
2. Halve and squeeze the limes. Put the meat cubes on the wooden skewers.
3. Mix together paprika powder, cayenne pepper, 3 tbsp lime juice, tamarind pulp and ketchup.
4. Turn meat skewers in it, cover with cling film, and leave to stand in the refrigerator for at least 2 hours (marinate).
5. In the meantime, wash and quarter the tomatoes, cutting out the stalks. Core the tomatoes and cut each quarter in half crosswise.
6. Peel and roughly dice the onions. Halve the pepper, remove the core, wash carefully and finely chop.
7. Halve the avocados, remove the stones. Lift the pulp out of the skin with a spoon and cut into large cubes.
8. Wash the coriander, shake dry, pluck the leaves and chop.
9. Mix with 1 tbsp lime juice, tomatoes, onions, pepper and avocado, season with salt and pepper.
10. Grill the skewers in a grill pan or over charcoal over medium heat for 7-8 minutes.
11. Serve with avocado and tomato salad.

Nutritional Value per Serving

312 Kcal	16 g Fat	13g Carbs	26g Protein	4.5 g Fiber	4g Added Sugar

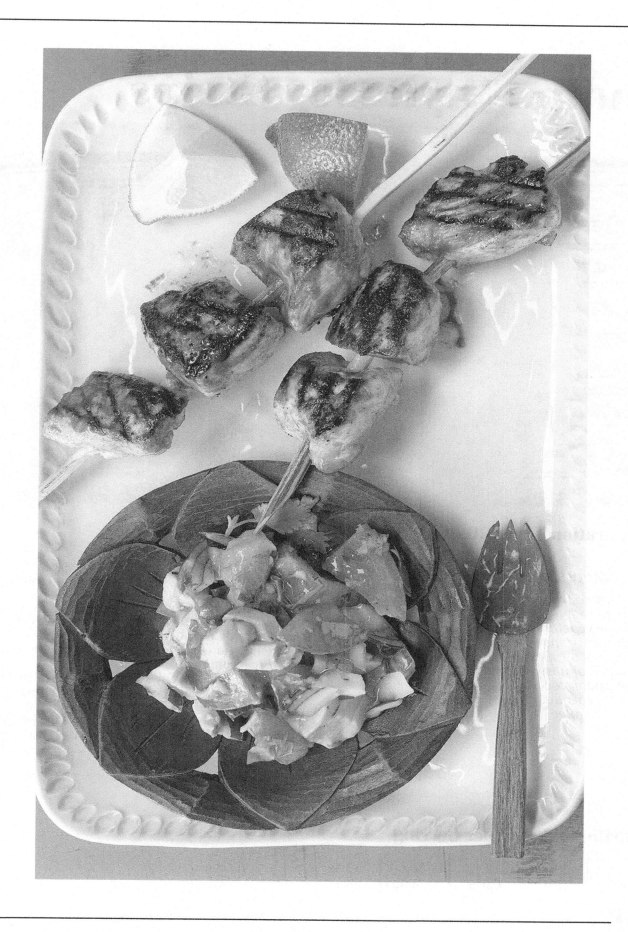

Indian-Style Soy Strips

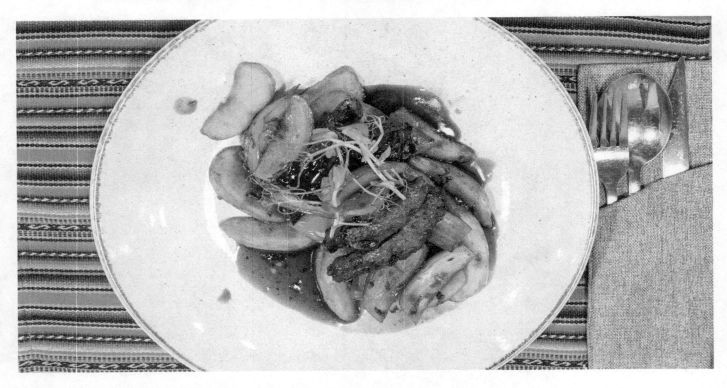

Preparation Time: 20 min

Ingredients for 3 people:

- 150 g soy strips
- 300 ml vegetable stock
- 1 large vegetable onion
- 1 tbsp curry powder
- 1 teaspoon rapeseed oil
- 2 halves of unsweetened (canned) peaches
- 1 teaspoon coconut oil
- 200 ml coconut milk
- Salt & pepper

1. Put the soy strips in a bowl and pour the hot vegetable stock over them to cover.
2. Let it soak for 15 to 20 minutes.
3. Meanwhile, cut the onions into rings, sweat them in oil and dust them with plenty of curry.
4. Briefly sauté the chopped peaches, then remove everything from the pan.
5. Drain the soaked soy strips, fry them in coconut oil (this takes a while due to the moisture content), sprinkle with curry and deglaze with the coconut milk.
6. Add the onion and peach mixture again, bring to the boil again and season to taste with curry, salt and pepper.

Nutritional Value per Serving

211 Kcal	6 g Fat	12.1g Carbs	26g Protein	13.4g Fiber

Pointed Cabbage in Soy Cream with Paprika Seasoning

Preparation Time: 25 min

Ingredients for 2 people:

- 300 g small pointed cabbage (1/2 small pointed cabbage)
- 2 small onions
- 1 tbsp rapeseed oil
- 1 tbsp paprika powder (noble sweet)
- 150 ml soy cream
- 100 ml classic vegetable broth
- 3 stems dill
- salt & pepper

1. Clean and wash the pointed cabbage, if necessary, remove the stalk in a wedge shape and cut the cabbage into fine strips. Peel the onions and cut them into fine strips.
2. Heat the oil in a saucepan and sauté the onions over medium heat until translucent.
3. Add the pointed cabbage and cook for another 3 minutes.
4. Sprinkle with paprika powder, pour in soy cream and broth.
5. Cook for 8-10 minutes over medium heat.
6. In the meantime, wash the dill, shake it dry, pluck off the flags and chop finely.
7. At the end of the cooking time, season the cabbage with salt and pepper and mix in the dill.

Nutritional Value per Serving

208 Kcal	18 g Fat	5g Carbs	5g Protein	4g Fiber	1g Added Sugar

Indian Vegetable Spiced Rice With Mango Chutney Yogurt

Preparation Time: 50 min

Ingredients for 4 people:

- 200 g basmati rice
- 1 tbsp turmeric
- Salt & pepper
- 50 g sultanas
- 75 g almond kernels
- 30 g ginger (1 piece)
- 3 garlic cloves
- 125 g onions (2 onions)
- 150 g spinach leaves
- 500 g zucchini (2 zucchini)
- 200 g carrots (2 carrots)
- 3 tbsp oil
- 5 cardamom pods
- 2 cloves
- 8 black peppercorns
- 1 tbsp garam masala
- 1 tbsp ground coriander
- 1 tsp cumin
- 250 ml classic vegetable broth
- 125 g mango chutney (5 tbsp)
- 300 g yogurt (0.3% fat)

1. Rinse rice with cold water and drain. Cook rice with turmeric in boiling salted water for 20 minutes over low heat, drain and set aside.
2. While the rice is cooking, soak the sultanas in hot water.
3. Roughly chop the almonds. Peel the ginger and grate finely. Peel and mash the garlic.
4. Grate the almonds with ginger and garlic in a mortar to a fine paste.
5. Peel the onions and cut them into fine cubes. Clean the spinach, wash thoroughly, drain well and roughly chop.
6. Wash the zucchini, rub dry and cut into 5 mm cubes. Wash and peel the carrots and cut them into 5 mm thin slices.
7. Heat the oil in a saucepan and steam the onions in it, stirring, until they are light brown.
8. Add cardamom, cloves and peppercorns and sauté briefly.
9. Add almond paste and stir-fry for 2 minutes.
10. Add the carrots, zucchini, garam masala, coriander and cumin, sauté briefly and pour in the broth.
11. Cover the vegetables and cook for 2-3 minutes.
12. Squeeze the sultanas, add to the saucepan with the spinach and rice and stir.
13. Cook covered for 4-5 minutes over medium heat, stirring twice.
14. Season the seasoned vegetable rice with salt and pepper.
15. Mix the mango chutney and yogurt and serve with the rice.

Nutritional Value per Serving

515 Kcal	19 g Fat	68g Carbs	14g Protein	10g Fiber	6g Add Sugar

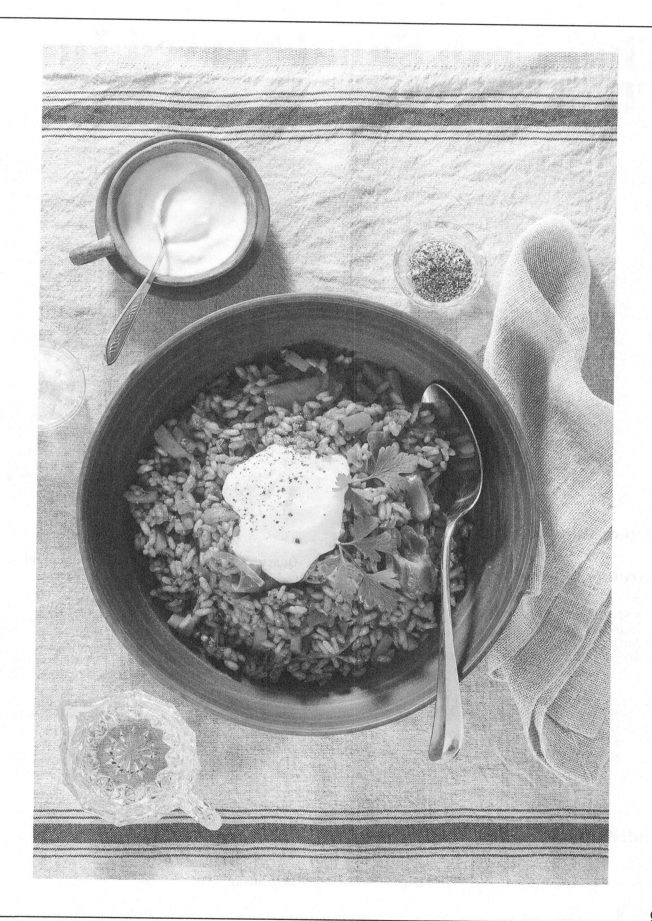

Thai Crab Salad Served In The Papaya

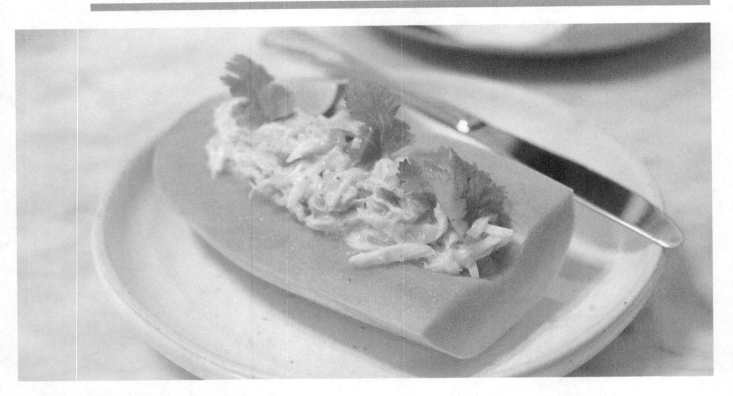

Preparation Time: 30 min

Ingredients for 4 people:

- 300 g small peppers (1 red, 1 green, 2 small peppers)
- 350 g crab meat
- 1 large shallot
- 1 kg small papaya (3 small papayas)
- 30 g ginger (1 piece)
- 1 red chili pepper
- 2 tbsp rice vinegar
- 3 tbsp Thai fish sauce
- 1 tbsp sugar
- ¼ tsp salt
- ½ fret coriander

1. Quarter, core, wash and cut the peppers into 5 mm cubes.
2. Peel and finely chop shallot.
3. Peel and core 1 papaya and cut into 5 mm cubes.
4. Peel the ginger, cut into pieces and squeeze in a garlic press, collect the juice. Halve, core, wash and finely chop the chili pepper.
5. Mix the ginger juice, vinegar, fish sauce, sugar, salt and 2 tablespoons of water until the sugar and salt have dissolved.
6. Examine the crab meat for any shell fragments.
7. Gently mix all the prepared ingredients in a bowl.
8. Wash the coriander, shake dry, pluck the leaves, but leave the tender stems on the leaves.
9. Halve the remaining papayas and remove the seeds. Line the papaya halves with the coriander and fill in the salad.
10. Serve immediately.

Nutritional Value per Serving

146 Kcal	2 g Fat	12g Carbs	19g Protein	6g Fiber	5g Added Sugar

84

Stewed Cucumbers with Salmon and Dill

Preparation Time: 20 min

Ingredients for 2 people:

- *500 g cucumber (1 cucumber)*
- *1 red onion*
- *250 g salmon fillet (125 g each)*
- *1 tbsp*
- *olive oil*
- *salt & pepper*
- *100 ml classic vegetable broth*
- *100 g sour cream (10% fat)*
- *1 bunch*
- *dill*
- *30 g sunflower seeds (2 tbsp)*

1. Clean the cucumber, peel and cut in half. Scrape out the seeds with a teaspoon. Cut the cucumber into pieces about 1.5 cm wide.
2. Peel and chop the onion.
3. Rinse the salmon fillet, pat dry and cut into 2 cm cubes.
4. Heat the oil in a pan and fry the fish in it for 4 minutes over medium heat until light brown.
5. Take out, season with salt and pepper.
6. Put the onion cubes in the hot pan and sauté for 2 minutes over medium heat.
7. Add the cucumber and cook for 2 minutes. Season with salt and pepper.
8. Add the stock and sour cream, bring to the boil briefly and then simmer over low heat for 4–5 minutes.
9. Meanwhile, wash the dill, shake it dry and chop it. Return the salmon to the pan.
10. Cook for another 2 minutes, season with salt and pepper. S
11. Serve sprinkled with dill and sunflower seeds.

Nutritional Value per Serving

527 Kcal	38 g Fat	14g Carbs	33g Protein	4.1 g Fiber	0g Added Sugar

Brazilian Fish Pot With Coconut And Chili

Preparation Time: 45 mins

Ingredients for 4 people:

- 400 g white fish fillet (monkfish, cod or halibut)
- 1 bunch spring onions as desired
- 200 g prawns (without head and shell)
- 150 g onions (3 onions)
- 4 garlic cloves
- 1 small red pepper
- 1 small yellow pepper
- 1 small green pepper
- 2 red chili peppers
- 400 g tomatoes (5 tomatoes)
- 1 rod celery
- 2 tbsp oil
- Salt & pepper
- 1 piece ginger to taste
- 200 ml coconut water
- 1 l poultry broth
- 1 tbsp ground cumin
- 1 lime
- 1 bunch coriander

1. Peel the onions and garlic. Finely dice the onions, cut the garlic into fine slices.
2. Halve, core and wash the peppers. Cut the peppers into 1 cm cubes. Wash the chill peppers, cut in half lengthways and core. Finely chop the chili peppers.
3. Wash the tomatoes, cut out the stalks in a wedge shape. Quarter and core the tomatoes. Wash and clean celery and, if necessary, remove threads and cut into cubes.
4. Heat the oil in a large saucepan. Sauté the onions, garlic, paprika and celery cubes over medium heat for 4–5 minutes while stirring. Add tomatoes and chili and cook for 1 minute. Salt and pepper. Finely chop ginger to taste and add.
5. Pour in coconut water and stock, season with cumin and bring to a boil. Cook on low heat for 10 minutes.
6. In the meantime, squeeze 3 tablespoons of juice from the lime. Wash the coriander, shake dry and pluck the leaves off. Pat the fish dry and cut it into large pieces. Wash and clean the spring onions as desired and cut them into thin slices.
7. Put the prawns in the pot, then add the pieces of fish and cook covered for 5 minutes over low heat.
8. Season the stew with lime juice and sprinkle with coriander.
9. If desired, serve the spring onions separately with the Brazilian fish pot.

Nutritional Value per Serving

280 Kcal	7 g Fat	15g Carbs	34g Protein	7g Fiber	0g Add Sugar

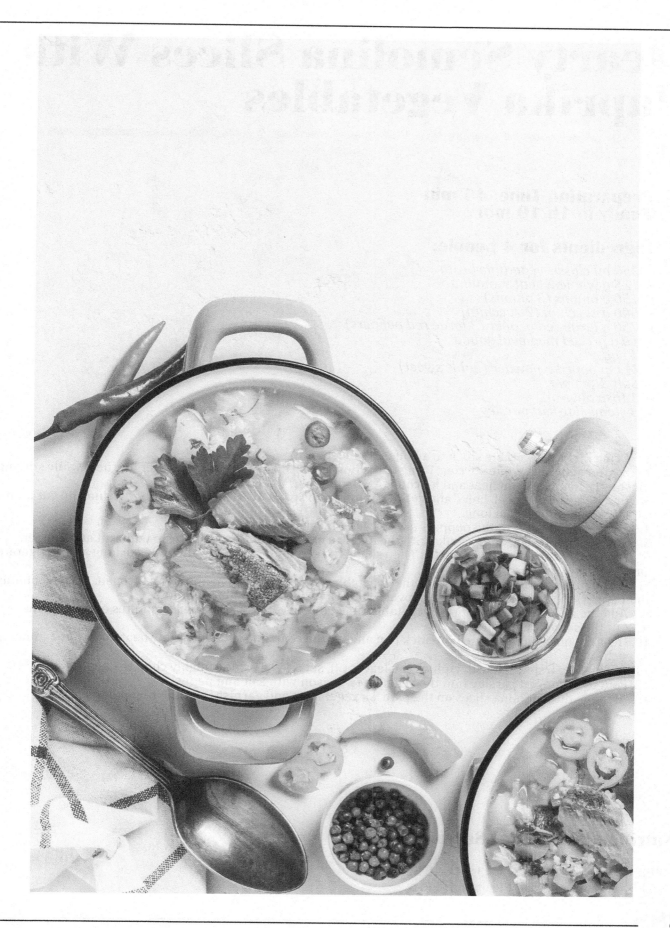

Hearty Semolina Slices With Paprika Vegetables

Preparation Time: 45 min
Ready in 1h 10 min

Ingredients for 4 people:

- *350 ml classic vegetable broth*
- *125 g whole wheat semolina*
- *150 g onions (3 onions)*
- *500 g zucchini (2 zucchini)*
- *750 g large red pepper (3 large red peppers)*
- *50 g grated medieval gouda*
- *1 egg*
- *½ tsp paprika powder (noble sweet)*
- *Salt & pepper*
- *1 tbsp olive oil*
- *3 stems flat-leaf parsley*

1. Bring 250 ml vegetable stock to a boil in a saucepan.
2. Scatter semolina while stirring, bring to the boil and let swell for 2 minutes over low heat while stirring constantly. Remove from heat and let cool for 10 minutes.
3. In the meantime, peel, halve and cut the onions into strips. Wash and clean the zucchini and cut it into narrow strips about 5 cm long.
4. Halve, core and wash the peppers and cut lengthways into strips.
5. Stir the cheese, egg and paprika into the lukewarm semolina. Season to taste with salt and pepper.
6. Dampen a work board with water. Then shape the semolina into a roll about 24 cm long and refrigerate for 10 minutes.
7. In the meantime, bring the rest of the vegetable stock to the boil in another saucepan. Add the onions and peppers, bring to a boil and cook covered over low heat for about 10 minutes.
8. Add the zucchini to the paprika vegetables and cook covered for another 4 minutes over low heat.
9. Cut the semolina roll into 12 slices.
10. Heat the olive oil in a large non-stick pan and fry the semolina slices over low heat for about 2 minutes on each side.
11. Rinse the parsley, shake dry, pluck the leaves off, set a third aside, roughly chop the rest.
12. Fold the chopped parsley into the vegetables, season with salt and pepper.
13. Arrange the semolina slices on the paprika vegetables and garnish with the remaining parsley.

Nutritional Value per Serving

295 Kcal	9 g Fat	30g Carbs	13g Protein	10.5g Fiber

Salmon Cutlet On Kohlrabi Salad With Fennel and Watercress

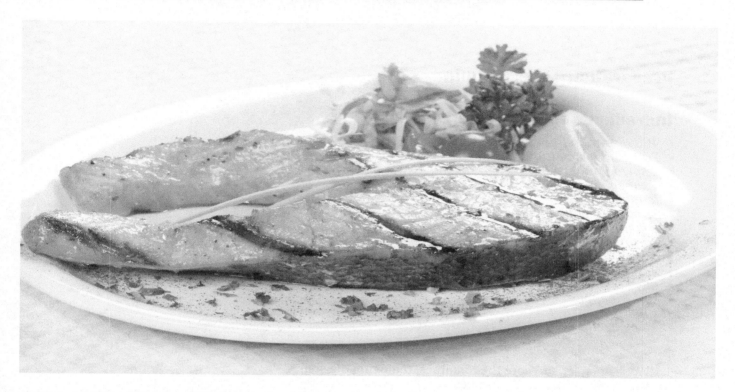

Preparation Time: 25 min

Ingredients for 2 people:

- *1 small shallot*
- *200 g small kohlrabi (1 small kohlrabi)*
- *1 tuber*
- *fennel*
- *50 g watercress*
- *200 g thin salmon cutlet (2 thin salmon cutlets)*
- *pepper*
- *4 tsp olive oil*
- *iodized salt with fluoride*
- *3 tbsp apple cider vinegar*
- *½ tsp mustard*
- *1 tsp liquid honey*

1. Peel and finely dice the shallot. Put in a fine sieve and scald with boiling water.
2. Peel and clean the kohlrabi, wash and clean the fennel. Cut both into small cubes.
3. Wash watercress and shake dry, cut into bite-sized pieces as desired.
4. Rinse the salmon cutlets, pat dry, season with pepper.
5. Heat 2 teaspoons of oil in a coated pan. Fry the salmon cutlets on each side for 3-4 minutes and lightly salt.
6. Mix vinegar, mustard, honey and remaining oil in a small bowl.
7. Mix the kohlrabi, fennel, shallot and watercress with the sauce.
8. Serve with the salmon cutlets.

Nutritional Value per Serving

334 Kcal	22 g Fat	9g Carbs	23g Protein	3.5 g Fiber	1g Added Sugar

Grilled Salmon Skewers with Fennel and Tomato Salsa

Preparation Time: 40 min

Ingredients for 4 people:

- *400 g salmon fillet without skin*
- *200 g fully ripe tomatoes*
- *2 spring onions*
- *1 tuber*
- *fennel*
- *1 red chili pepper*
- *3 stems*
- *coriander*
- *1 lime*
- *3 tbsp*
- *olive oil*
- *salt & pepper*
- *sugar*
- *1 dried chili pepper*

1. Wash, quarter and core the tomatoes, removing the stalks.
2. Divide the pulp into 1 cm cubes.
3. Wash and clean the spring onions and cut into rings 1/2 cm thick.
4. Wash the fennel, cut in half, remove the stalk and finely dice the tuber.
5. Halve the fresh chili lengthways, remove the core, wash and finely chop.
6. Wash the coriander, shake dry and chop the leaves.
7. Squeeze the lime.
8. Mix the finely chopped ingredients with 1 tablespoon each of lime juice and oil. Season with salt and a pinch of sugar.
9. Chill before serving and let steep for at least 30 minutes.
10. Cut the salmon fillet into 12 equal cubes.
11. Crumble the dried chili pepper, mix with the pepper and the remaining oil and pour over the salmon. Let it steep for 15 minutes (marinate).
12. Lightly salt the salmon cubes and place them on 4 wooden skewers.
13. Heat a grill pan and grill the skewers all around for 4-5 minutes.
14. Place the salmon skewers and salsa on a plate and serve with lime wedges if desired

Nutritional Value per Serving

225 Kcal	14 g Fat	4g Carbs	19g Protein	2.5 g Fiber	1g Added Sugar

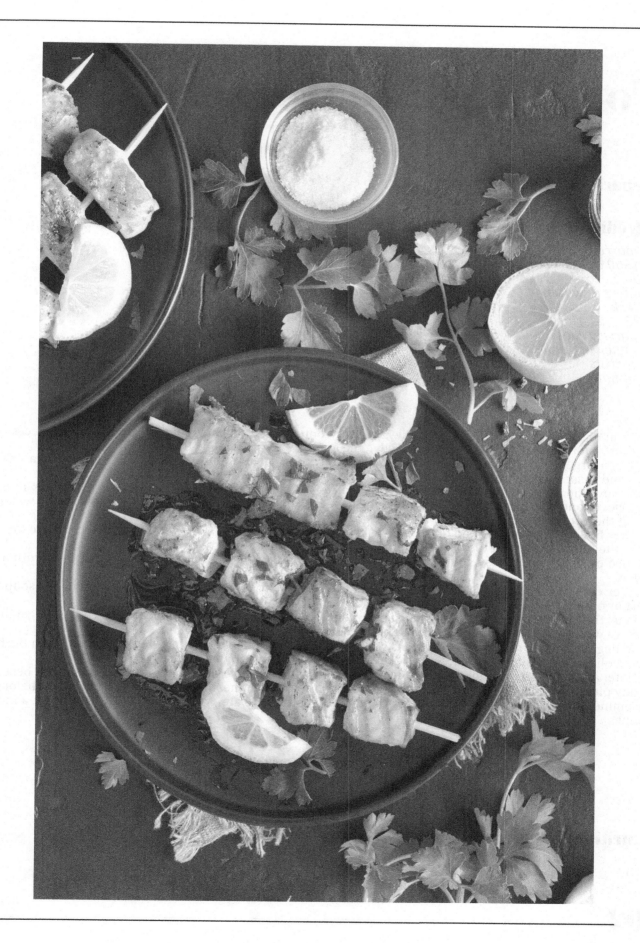

Fortifying Meat Broth

Preparation Time: 60 min

Ingredients for 2 - 2½ l stock:

- 3 marrow bones
- 2 (500 g each) beef leg slices
- 500 g oxtail
- 3 liters of water
- 1 leek
- 125 g celeriac
- 1 parsley root
- 1 bunch of parsley
- 2 carrots
- 1 tomato

- 2 onions
- 2 cloves of garlic
- 2 bay leaves
- 1 tbsp peppercorns
- 5 cloves
- 5 allspice grains
- a few sprigs of fresh thyme
- alternatively: 1 tbsp dried thyme
- 1 tbsp salt

1. Clean and wash the leek, celery, parsley, parsley root and carrots and roughly cut into small pieces. Wash tomatoes, cut in half and cut out the stalk. Halve the onions without peeling them.
2. Heat a large, tall saucepan without any fat. Place the onion halves in the saucepan with the cut surfaces facing down and roast them dry over medium to high heat until they are brown.
3. Remove the pan from the stove, add the bones, slices of leg and oxtail, sprinkle prepared vegetables, unpeeled garlic cloves and spices over it and fill up with cold water. The meat should be completely covered by water.
4. Put the pot back on the stove and bring the soup to a boil. Salt.
5. After boiling, repeatedly skim off the rising brownish foam with the skimmer. Then switch back to low heat, put on the lid, cover, and let the broth simmer for about 1½ hours.
6. Turn off the stove, remove the meat from the broth and place it on a plate or a carving board with a juice groove.
7. After cooling, the meat can be detached from the bones, cut into small pieces and added to the soup as an insert or otherwise used.
8. Pour the broth through a fine kitchen sieve into another pot and carefully squeeze the cooked vegetables in the sieve with a spoon or potato masher so that the juice gets into the broth.
9. To degrease the broth when the broth is still hot, pull layers of kitchen paper over the film of fat on the broth. After cooling, degreasing is easier: Simply lift off the solidified layer of fat with a flat trowel.
10. Note: A good broth is made with a long, gentle simmer. Expensive fillet meat does not make the best soup; streaky pieces such as ribs or slices of the leg are more suitable. Bones (marrow bones, oxtail) also belong in a consommé - they provide protein. For a broth of about 3 liters of water, you need about 1 kg of meat and 500 g of bones.

Nutritional Value per Serving

52 Kcal	3 g Fat	0.5g Carbs	6g Protein

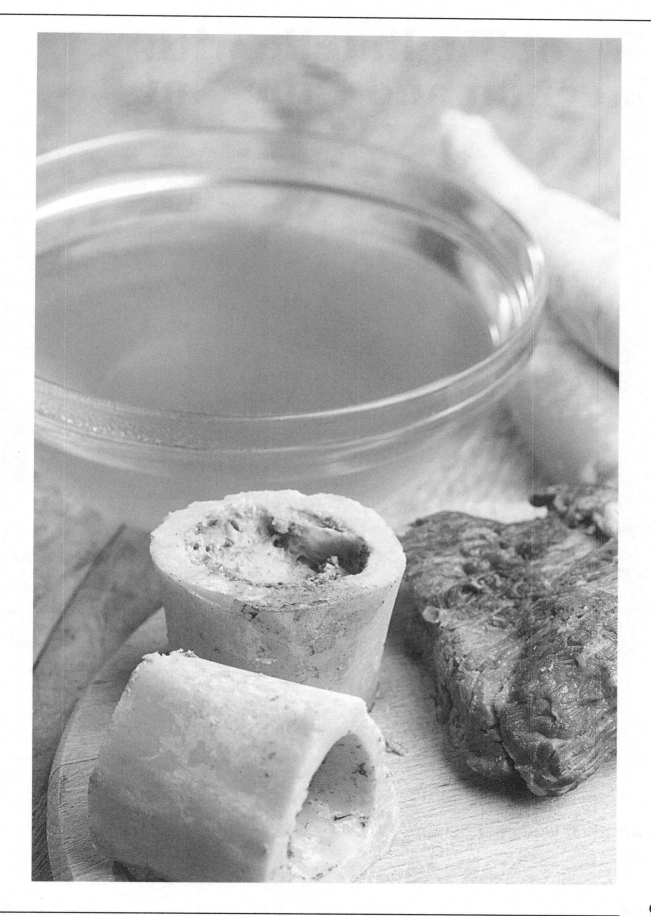

Carrot Tagliatelle with Zucchini and Pine Nuts

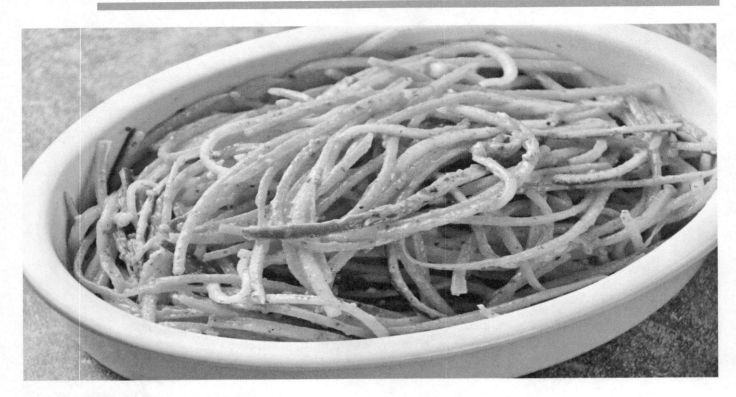

Preparation Time: 10 min

Ingredients for 2 people:

- 300 g Carrots
- 1 medium-size Zucchini
- 40 g Pine nuts
- 1 tbsp Olive oil
- Salt & pepper
- as desired: parsley or thyme

1. Clean and wash the carrots and use a vegetable peeler to slice them into thin strips - similar to ribbon noodles. Wash and clean the zucchini and cut it into bite-sized pieces.
2. Roast the pine nuts in a coated pan without fat until they smell and set aside.
3. Heat the olive oil in the pan, fry the zucchini pieces in it.
4. Season with salt, pepper and herbs to taste.
5. Meanwhile, bring water to a boil with a bit of salt in a medium-sized saucepan.
6. Blanch the carrot strips in it for 2 minutes. Rinse with cold water and drain in a colander.
7. Then add to the zucchini and toss briefly.
8. Distribute on preheated plates and sprinkle with the pine nuts.

Nutritional Value per Serving

218 Kcal	16 g Fat	12g Carbs	8g Protein	6 g Fiber

Baked Chicken Breast With Spinach and Sheep Cheese

Preparation Time: 25 min

Ingredients for 4 people:

- *450 g frozen spinach leaves*
- *4 (approx. 150 g each) chicken breast fillets*
- *100 g sheep cheese*
- *1 onion*
- *Salt & pepper*
- *freshly grated nutmeg*
- *2 teaspoons sesame oil or rapeseed oil*

1. Pre-heat the oven to 220 degrees Celsius.
2. Thaw the spinach.
3. In the meantime, wash the chicken breast fillets, pat dry and season generously with salt and pepper on both sides.
4. Heat 1 teaspoon of oil in a pan (be careful, it mustn't smoke!) And fry the chicken briefly on both sides.
5. Peel the onion and cut it into fine cubes. Heat the remaining oil in the pan and sauté the onion in it.
6. Briefly pre-cook the spinach in it, remove from the heat and season with salt, pepper and nutmeg.
7. Place the fried chicken breast fillets in a baking dish and spread the spinach on top.
8. Cut the sheep's cheese into cubes and sprinkle on top.
9. Bake everything in the oven on the middle rack for about 25 minutes.
10. Take out and let cool briefly before serving.

Nutritional Value per Serving

310 Kcal	14 g Fat	3g Carbs	43g Protein	3g Fiber

Bulgur Salad

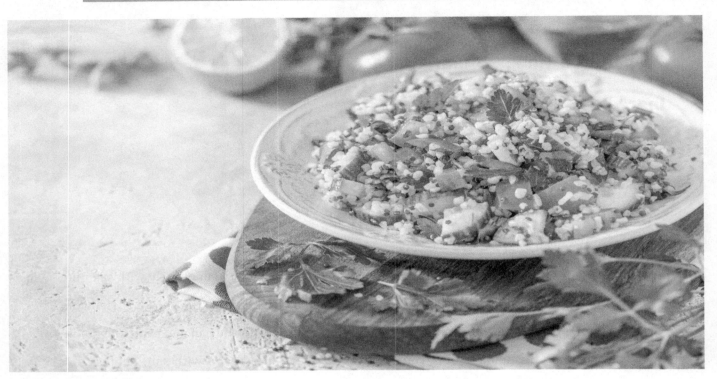

Preparation Time: 15 min

Ingredients for 4 people:

- 200 g of coarse bulgur
- 400 ml vegetable stock
- 250 g cucumber
- 2 beefsteak tomatoes
- 2 carrots
- 1 bunch of flat-leaf parsley
- 1 sprig of mint
- Salt & pepper
- nutmeg

Ingredients for the dressing:

- 4 tbsp olive oil
- 1 tbsp light balsamic vinegar
- Salt & pepper
- sugar
- cumin

1. Roast the bulgur in a hot saucepan without fat for about 1 minute.
2. Pour in the broth, bring to a boil, cover, and leave to soak for 15 minutes over low heat.
3. Let cool down, stirring several times.
4. In the meantime, wash the cucumber and cut it into small cubes.
5. Wash the tomatoes, cut in half and cut into small cubes, removing the pips and stems.
6. Clean, peel and finely grate the carrot.
7. Wash the parsley and mint and shake dry, pluck the leaves and chop finely.

1. For the vinaigrette, mix the vinegar in a bowl with salt, pepper and a pinch of sugar and cumin. Then hide the oil.
2. Mix the cooled bulgur with the vegetables and herbs in a large bowl and stir in the vinaigrette. To serve, season the salad with salt, pepper and nutmeg.

Nutritional Value per Seving

340 Kcal	15 g Fat	41g Carbs	6g Protein	8 g Fiber

Vegetable Curry with Red Lentils And Mango

Preparation Time: 15 min

Ingredients for 4 people:

- *80 g red lentils*
- *1 can (400 ml) organic coconut milk*
- *400 ml of water*
- *1 onion*
- *1 finger-thick piece of ginger*
- *2 cloves of garlic*
- *2 zucchinis*
- *1 red pepper*
- *1 yellow pepper*
- *2 carrots*
- *1 mango*
- *1 tbsp coconut oil*
- *1 tbsp tomato paste*
- *1 tbsp curry*
- *1 tbsp turmeric*
- *Salt & pepper*

1. Peel and finely chop the onion, ginger and garlic.
2. Clean and wash the remaining vegetables and cut them into bite-sized pieces.
3. Rinse and drain the lentils in a colander.
4. Heat the coconut oil and briefly fry the vegetables in it.
5. Add the lentils and ginger and toast them briefly.
6. Pour coconut milk and water on top.
7. Add tomato paste and the remaining spices and simmer covered for about 15 minutes over medium heat.
8. Meanwhile, peel the mango with the peeler, cut the pulp from the stone and dice.
9. Pour over the finished vegetable curry and serve.

Nutritional Value per Serving

165 Kcal	4g Fat	23g Carbs	8g Protein	8g Fiber

Couscous with Chicken

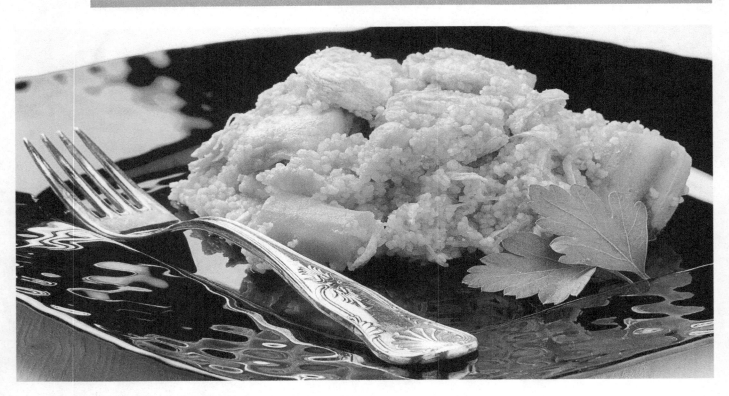

Preparation Time: 16 min

Ingredients for 4 people:

- 4 (125 g each) chicken fillets
- 2 cloves of garlic
- 4 onions
- 4 carrots
- 1/2 (approx. 200 g) celeriac
- 2 tbsp olive oil
- 100 g couscous
- 600 ml vegetable stock
- little salt & pepper
- coriander
- Caraway seed
- 6 stalks of parsley

1. Wash the chicken breast fillets, pat dry, and cut into cubes. Peel the garlic and onions and cut both into fine cubes. Clean and peel the carrots and celery and also cut them into cubes.
2. Heat the oil in a large saucepan and sauté the chicken all over. Add the vegetables and cook for about 6 minutes. Then add the couscous and sauté briefly. Deglaze with broth and cook for about 10 minutes.
3. In the meantime, wash the parsley and shake dry, pluck the leaves and chop finely.
4. Season the couscous with a bit of salt, pepper, coriander and caraway seeds, distribute on plates and serve sprinkled with parsley.

Nutritional Value per Serving

380 Kcal	11 g Fat	29g Carbs	36g Protein	8g Fiber

Herb Omelet with Smoked Salmon

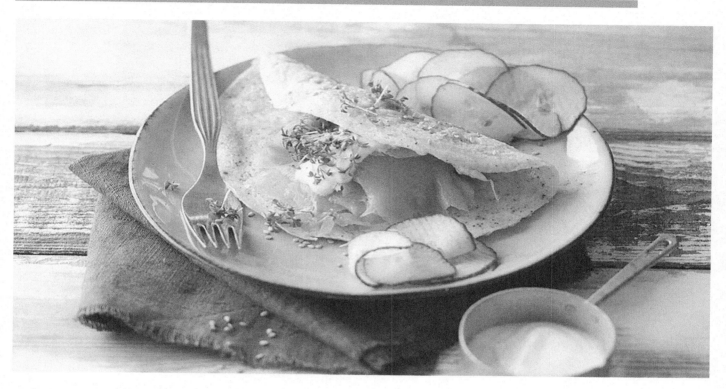

Preparation Time: 20 mins

Ingredients for 2 people:

- *300 g cucumber*
- *50 g smoked salmon*
- *1 box of garden cress*
- *3 eggs*
- *2 tbsp mineral water*
- *Salt & pepper*
- *2 tbsp kefir*
- *2 tbsp freshly chopped dill*
- *2 tbsp chives rolls*
- *2 tbsp rapeseed oil*

1. Wash or peel the cucumber and cut diagonally into thin slices, lay out flat on plates and sprinkle with salt. Cut the salmon into cubes. Cut the cress from the bed, wash and pat dry.
2. Whisk the eggs with salt, pepper, mineral water and kefir. Fold in the dill and chives. Heat the oil in a pan, add the egg mixture and let it set over low heat to make an omelet.
3. Sprinkle with salmon cubes and cress. Fold, cut in half and arrange on the cucumber slices. Serve immediately.

Nutritional Value per Serving

320 Kcal	24 g Fat	5g Carbs	18g Protein	2g Fiber

Soups

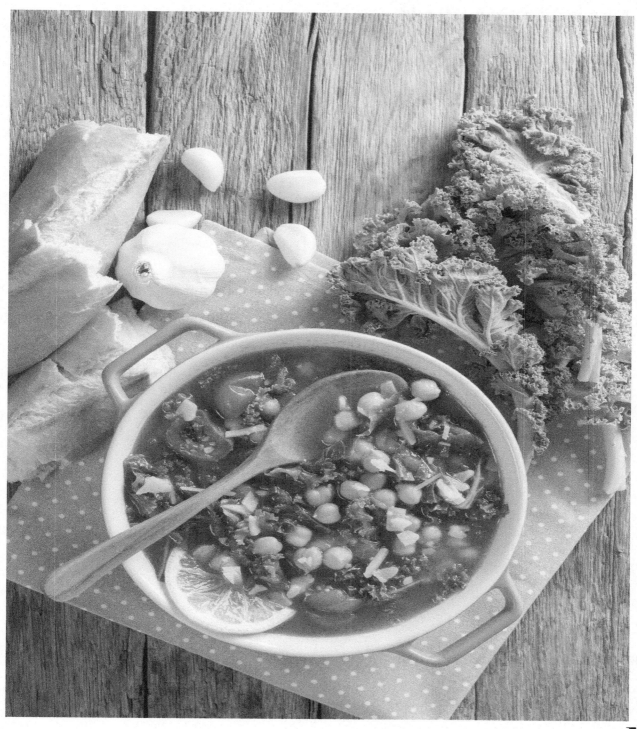

Red Lentil Soup With Basil Gremolata

Preparation Time: 10 min

Ingredients per 2 people

- *170 g red lentils*
- *1 onion*
- *1 clove of garlic*
- *1 carrot*
- *5 sun-dried tomatoes*
- *2 tbsp olive oil*
- *800 ml of water*
- *1 teaspoon sea salt*
- *1 teaspoon almond butter*
- *alternatively: 1 tbsp ground almonds*
- *2 tbsp lime juice*
- *1 teaspoon grated lime zest*
- *black pepper*
- *½ pot of basil*

1. Peel and roughly chop the onion and clove of garlic. Peel the carrot and cut it into cubes. Drain the sun-dried tomatoes on paper towels.
2. Heat the olive oil in a medium saucepan. Sweat the onion, garlic and carrot in it for 3 minutes while stirring.
3. Meanwhile, rinse the lentils thoroughly. Add the lentils, water and salt, bring to a boil.
4. Switch back to medium heat and cook the lentils with the lid closed for about 10 minutes.
5. For the gremolata, cut off the basil stalks, wash and shake dry. Wash the chili pepper, remove the seeds and separate membranes. Finely chop the chili, basil and 2 sun-dried tomatoes. Pour into a bowl, mix with the lime zest and 1 tbsp lime juice.
6. Puree the soup with the remaining sun-dried tomatoes and almond butter - if the consistency is too thick, add a little more water.
7. Season to taste with salt, pepper and the remaining lime juice.
8. Divide the soup on deep plates and place the gremolata in the middle.

Nutritional Value per Serving

470 Kcal	12 g Fat	50g Carbs	30g Protein	20 g Fiber

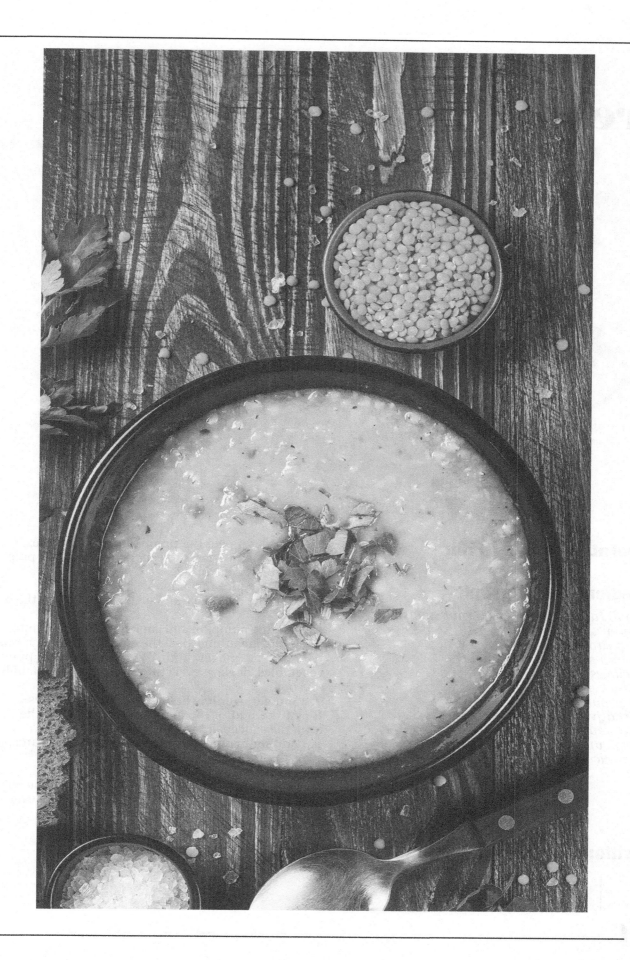

Cream Of Butternut Soup

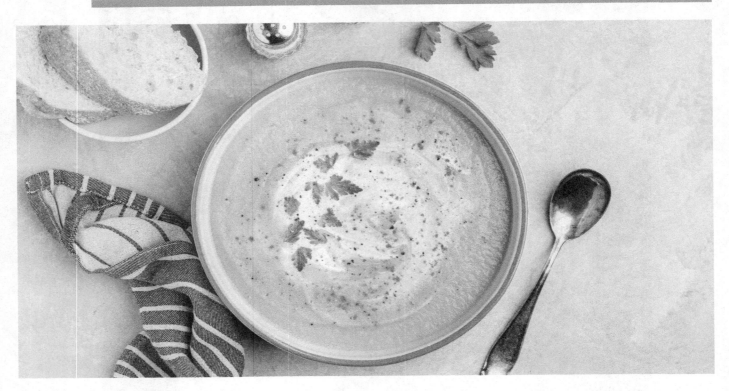

Preparation Time: 30 min

Ingredients for 4 people

- *1 small (approx. 1 kg) butternut squash*
- *1 onion*
- *2 tbsp rapeseed oil*
- *1 thumb-sized piece of ginger*
- *1-2 cloves*
- *600 ml vegetable stock*
- *100 g sour cream*
- *alternatively: 100 g sour cream*
- *salt & pepper*
- *4 tbsp pumpkin seed oil*
- *Turmeric powder*

1. Wash and peel the pumpkin, cut into slices, scrape out the seeds with a tablespoon and cut the pulp into pieces about 2 cm in size.
2. Peel and dice the onion.
3. Heat the oil in a large saucepan and sauté the onion in it.
4. Add the pumpkin and cook for about 5 minutes.
5. In the meantime, peel the ginger and grate it finely.
6. Add the ginger and 1-2 cloves to the pumpkin vegetables, deglaze everything with the stock and bring to a boil.
7. Simmer over low heat for about 30 minutes.
8. At the end of the cooking time, remove the cloves from the saucepan.
9. Add sour cream or sour cream to the soup and puree everything with the hand blender.
10. Season to taste with salt and pepper.
11. To serve, distribute on plates and refine with 1 tablespoon each of pumpkin seed oil (please never cook this fine oil) and 1 pinch of turmeric.

Nutritional Value per Serving

297 Kcal	26 g Fat	10g Carbs	3g Protein	7g Fiber

Asia Noodle Soup

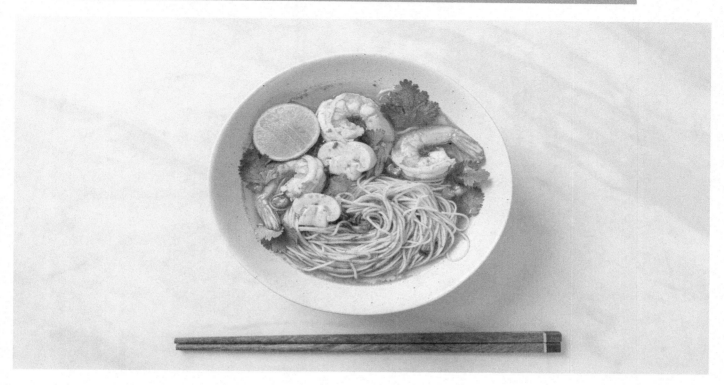

Preparation Time: 18 min

Ingredients for 2 people:

- 100 g radish
- 100 g Pak choi
- 30 g Rice noodles
- 200 g raw, peeled prawns
- 50 g Mung bean sprouts
- 700 ml gluten-free vegetable broth
- 0.5 fret Coriander green
- 10 g ginger
- 1 tbsp light sesame oil
- 1 tsp toasted sesame oil
- 2.5 tbsp (e.g., Tamari) soy sauce
- 0.5 tsp Five-spice powder

1. Peel and finely dice the ginger. Heat both types of sesame oil in a saucepan and sauté the ginger over medium heat for 1 to 2 minutes. Pour in the broth and slowly bring to a boil. Season with soy sauce and five-spice powder, simmer everything with the lid closed over low heat for about 10 minutes.
2. In the meantime, wash the prawns as needed and pat dry. Clean, wash and thinly slice the radishes. Clean the pak choi, remove the ends and stems and cut the leaves into strips 1 to 2 cm wide.
3. Add the vegetables and, if necessary, the prawns to the soup, bring everything to a boil and cook with the lid closed over medium heat for about 5 minutes. After about 3 minutes, add the rice noodles and cook at the same time.
4. Rinse and drain the sprouts in a sieve. Wash the coriander leaves, shake dry, pluck the leaves and roughly chop. To serve, divide the soup on deep plates and sprinkle with sprouts and coriander greens.

1. **Note:** *The soup can be prepared with or without prawns as you like.*

Nutritional Value per Serving without Shrimp

231 Kcal	14g Fat	19g Carbs	6g Protein	6g Fiber

Nutritional Value per Serving whit Shrimp

350 Kcal	17g Fat	21g Carbs	26g Protein	6 g Fiber

Tomato Soup Made From Fresh Tomatoes

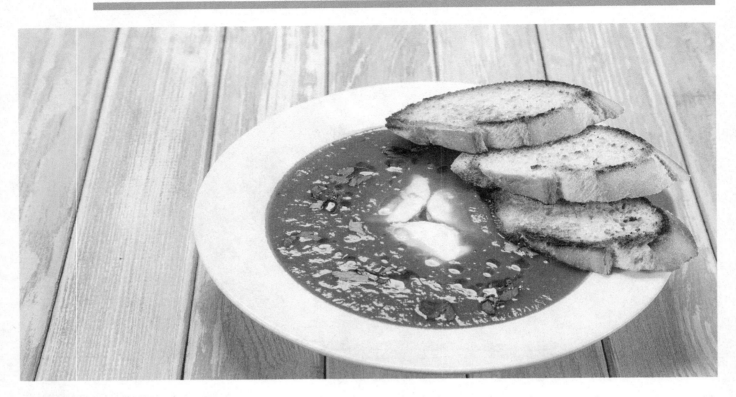

Preparation Time: 40 min

Ingredients for 2 people:

- 1 kg of tomatoes
- 200 ml of water
- ½ teaspoon salt
- 1 sprig of rosemary
- 1 sprig of thyme
- 2 tbsp heavy cream
- 2 tbsp sour cream

1. Whsh the tomatoes and put them in a saucepan with water and salt. Bring to a boil.
2. Simmer for 10-15 minutes, until the peel starts to peel off the tomatoes and the tomatoes are soft.
3. In the meantime, wash the herbs and let them dry on paper towels.
4. Drain the tomatoes, collecting the cooking water if necessary. Strain or strain the soft tomatoes through a sieve. Let the pureed tomatoes simmer for about 10 minutes.
5. Then stir with the cream until smooth. Dilute as desired with some of the collected cooking water.
6. Strip off the rosemary and thyme needles and chop finely.
7. Fill the soup into two bowls, put a dollop of sour cream on top and sprinkle everything with the herbs.

Nutritional Value per Serving

186 Kcal	8g Fat	21g Carbs	6g Protein	2 g Fiber

Pumpkin Soup With Ginger

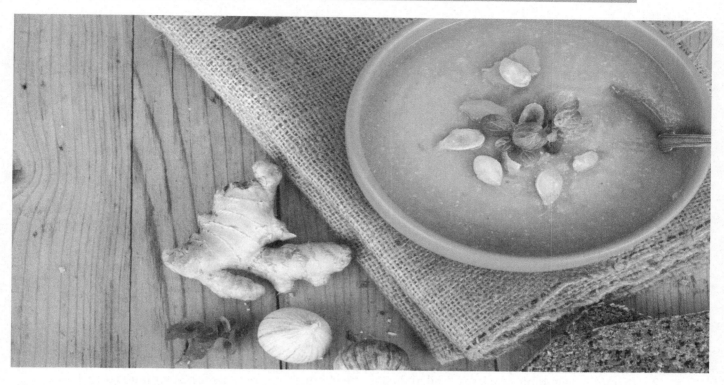

Preparation Time: 20 min

Ingredients per 2 people

- approx. 350 g Hokkaido pumpkin
- 2 cloves of garlic
- 2 medium onions
- 1 piece (approx. 5 cm) of ginger
- ½ tsp grained vegetable broth
- 1 tbsp rapeseed oil
- Curry powder
- 1-2 tbsp sour cream
- Pepper

1. Wash the Hokkaido pumpkin, cut it in half and remove the seeds and fibers with a spoon.
2. Cut the pumpkin flesh with the skin into cubes.
3. Peel the onion and garlic, cut the onion into large cubes and the garlic into fine cubes.
4. Peel and finely chop the ginger.
5. Mix the instant broth with 600 ml of boiling water.
6. Heat the oil in a large saucepan and sauté the onion in it. Add the garlic and ginger and sauté briefly. Dust with curry powder to taste and stir briefly. Then add the pumpkin cubes and brown all over while stirring.
7. Deglaze with the broth and cover and simmer over low heat for 15-20 minutes until the pumpkin is creamy. Stir occasionally.
8. Then stir in the sour cream and 100 ml of water. Puree everything finely with a hand blender and briefly bring to the boil again.
9. To serve, season the soup with fresh pepper from the mill and divide into deep plates.

Nutritional Value per Serving

220 Kcal	14 g Fat	14g Carbs	4g Protein	6 g Fiber	

Hawaiian Curry Soup

Preparation Time: 30 min

Ingredients for 4 people:

- *2 carrots*
- *1 leek*
- *1 apple*
- *1 onion*
- *1 clove of garlic*
- *1 piece (2 cm) of ginger*
- *1 l vegetable stock*
- *200 ml coconut milk*
- *1 tbsp curry*
- *Salt & pepper*
- *1 stalk of lemongrass*
- *for binding: some flour*
- *2 tbsp (Thai) basil*

1. Clean, wash and chop the carrots, leek and apple. Peel the ginger, onion and garlic and chop very finely.
2. Bring the vegetable stock to a boil and cook the chopped ingredients for 30 minutes until soft.
3. Add the coconut milk and puree the soup. Season to taste with salt, pepper and curry. Wash the lemongrass, add it to the soup, let it steep for ten minutes, and then remove it.
4. In a small bowl with a little water, stir the flour until smooth - the flour mixture must not be lumpy.
5. Stir into the soup to thicken, bring the soup to a boil again and stir vigorously.
6. Wash the (Thai) basil, shake it dry, chop it if necessary and garnish the soup with it.

Nutritional Value per Serving

100 Kcal	5g Fat	11g Carbs	2g Protein	4g Fiber

Beetroot Soup With Oranges

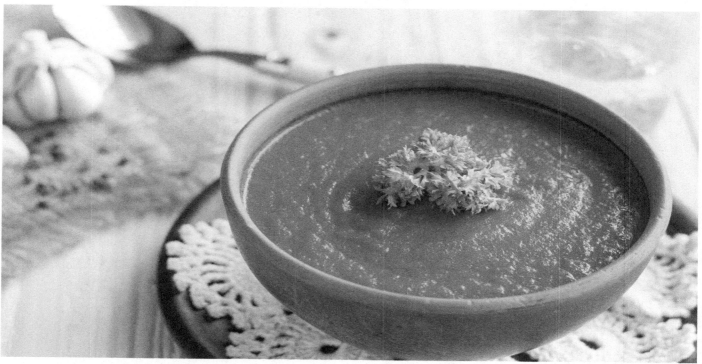

**Preparation Time: 40 min
Ready in 2h 20 min**

Ingredients for 4 people

- 600 g beetroot
- 3 shallots
- 2 juice oranges
- 2 tbsp rapeseed oil
- 800 ml classic vegetable broth
- 2 stems dill
- 125 ml soy cream
- Salt & pepper

1. Wash beetroot. Cut off the ends and wrap the vegetables one at a time in a piece of aluminum foil.
2. Bake in the preheated oven at 180 ° C (convection not recommended, gas: level 2-3) on the middle rack for 1 1/2 hours.
3. Take out the beetroot, let it cool down a bit and peel off the skin. (Work with gloves because of the color.)
4. In the meantime, peel and finely dice the shallots.
5. Peel the oranges with a knife so that all of the white skin is removed. Loosen the pulp from the separating membranes, catching the juice.
6. Squeeze the separating layers of the oranges in your hand and collect the juice.
7. Heat the oil in a saucepan and fry the shallot cubes in it over medium heat until translucent.
8. Cut the beetroot into small pieces and add. Simmer for 2 minutes.
9. Pour in the broth and add all of the orange juice.
10. Cook on medium heat for 15 minutes.
11. In the meantime, wash the dill, shake it dry and pluck the flags off.
12. Add half of the orange fillets to the beetroot soup and puree the soup finely.
13. Pour in the soy cream and briefly bring it to a boil again.
14. Season with salt and pepper.
15. Put the beetroot soup in bowls and garnish with the remaining orange fillets and dill.

Nutritional Value per Serving

186 Kcal	10g Fat	17g Carbs	4g Protein	5.5g Fiber	0g Added Sugar

Cream Of Potato Soup With Marjoram

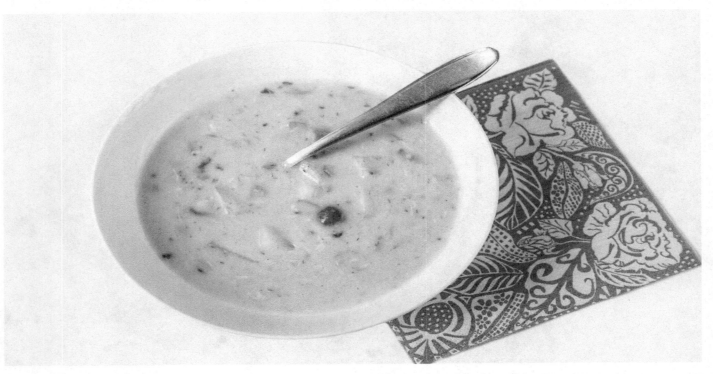

Preparation Time: 30 min

Ingredients for 2 people:

- 400 g mostly waxy potatoes
- 75 g kohlrabi
- 75 g zucchini
- 400 ml gluten-free vegetable stock
- 100 ml (from the tetra Pak) oat cream
- 2 sprigs of marjoram
- 1 bay leaf
- 1 small carrot
- 2 tablespoons of cold-pressed olive oil
- Salt & pepper
- freshly grated nutmeg

1. Peel, wash and dice the potatoes.
2. Heat ½ tbsp oil in a saucepan and simmer the potatoes in it over low heat for about 5 minutes. Season with pepper.
3. Pour in the stock and oat cream.
4. Wash the marjoram and add 1 sprig with the bay leaf to the soup.
5. Bring everything to a boil and cook with the lid closed over medium heat for about 20 minutes.
6. In the meantime, for the topping, clean and peel the carrot, kohlrabi and courgette or wash and dice very finely.
7. In a small pan, simmer in the rest of the oil over medium heat for about 5 minutes, turning.
8. Pluck the leaves from the remaining marjoram sprig, set some aside for garnish, and then finely chop the rest.
9. Add the marjoram to the vegetables, season with salt, pepper and nutmeg.
10. Remove the bay leaf and marjoram sprig from the soup and finely puree the soup with a hand blender.
11. Divide the soup on deep plates, sprinkle with diced vegetables and marjoram leaves.

Nutritional Value per Serving

360 Kcal	18g Fat	39g Carbs	6g Protein	5g Fiber

Potato Vegetable Soup

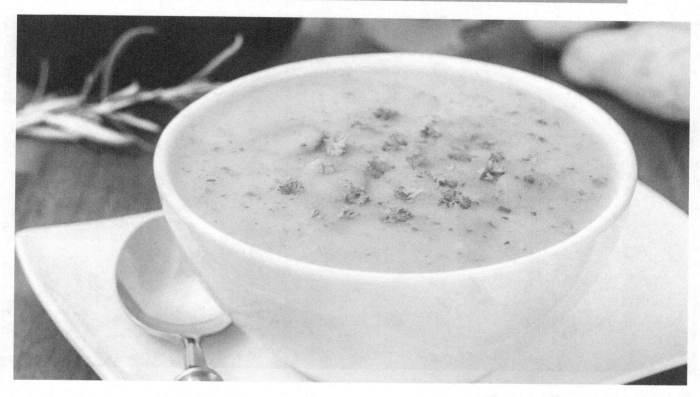

Preparation Time: 60 min

Ingredients per 2 people

- *150 g potatoes*
- *300 g vegetables*
- *1 tbsp rapeseed oil*
- *0.6 l of broth*
- *fresh thyme*
- *2 bay leaves*
- *pepper*

1. Peel the potatoes, clean the vegetables (e.g., zucchini, carrots, celery or fennel).
2. Cut everything into small pieces.
3. Carefully heat the oil in a saucepan.
4. Sauté the potatoes and vegetables for 2 minutes, then pour the stock and add the herbs.
5. Let everything simmer for about 10 minutes.
6. Fish out the bay leaves. Then puree the soup and season to taste again.

Nutritional Value per Serving

183 Kcal	10.8 g Fat	16.6g Carbs	5g Protein	5g Fiber

Tomato Soup With Zucchini Sticks

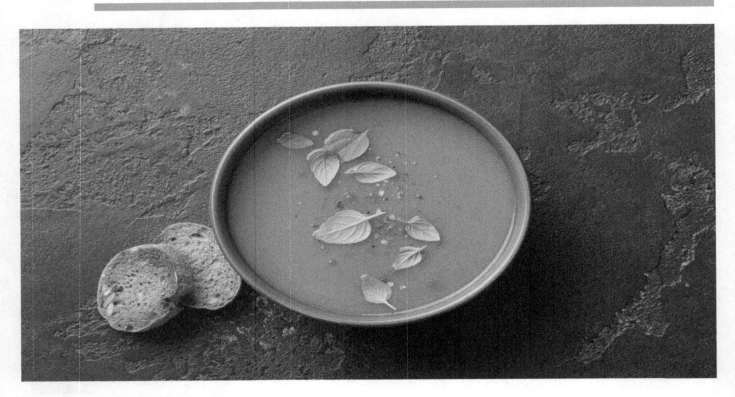

Preparation Time: 10 min

Ingredients for 2 people:

- *1 small onion*
- *2 cloves of garlic*
- *1 tbsp rapeseed oil*
- *1 can of tomatoes*
- *250 ml vegetable stock*
- *1 zucchini*
- *Salt & pepper*
- *Lemon juice*
- *2 tbsp sour cream*

1. Peel and finely dice the onion. Peel off the garlic cloves and chop finely.
2. Heat the oil in a pot. Fry the onion cubes and garlic slices until golden.
3. Add chunky tomatoes and vegetable stock, bring to a boil and simmer for 5 minutes over medium heat.
4. In the meantime, wash the zucchini and cut it into about 3 cm long, narrow sticks. Add to the soup and let simmer for another 5 minutes.
5. Season the soup with salt, pepper and lemon juice.
6. Divide between 2 plates and place 1 tbsp sour cream in the middle.

Nutritional Value per Serving

145 Kcal	9g Fat	10g Carbs	5g Protein

Parsnip and Potato Soup

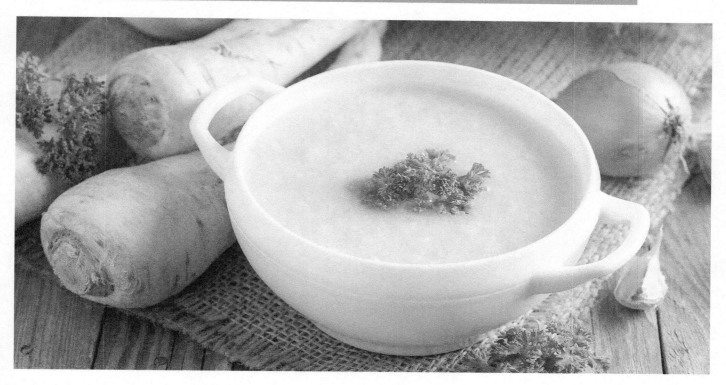

Preparation Time: 15 min

Ingredients for 4 people

- 300 g parsnips
- 300 g floury potatoes
- 2 tbsp olive oil
- 600 ml vegetable stock
- 200 ml (1 small can) coconut milk
- sea-salt
- from the mill: pepper
- 1 bunch of coriander or flat-leaf parsley

1. Peel, wash and dice parsnips and potatoes.
2. Heat the oil in a large saucepan and sweat the diced vegetables in it over medium to high heat for 2 minutes, stirring as you go.
3. Pour in the vegetable stock, bring to a boil and then cook over medium heat for about 15 minutes until soft.
4. Add the coconut milk and finely puree the soup with a hand blender.
5. Bring to the boil again briefly, season with salt and pepper and fill into preheated plates.
6. Finely chop the coriander or parsley and sprinkle over the soup.

Nutritional Value per Serving

156 Kcal	8g Fat	18g Carbs	2g Protein	3 g Fiber

Carrot Curry Soup

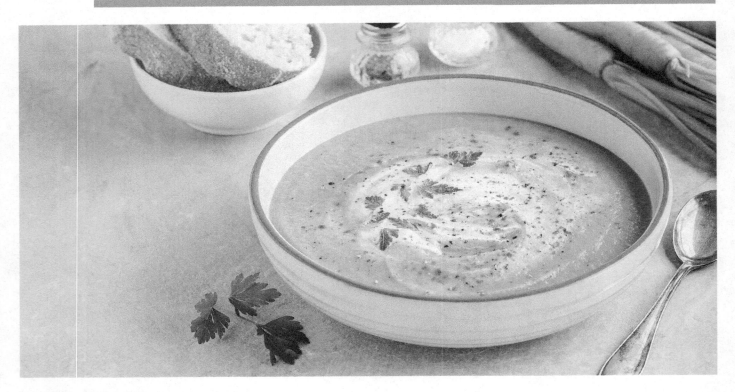

Preparation Time: 15 min

Ingredients for 4 people:

- approx. 300 g floury potatoes
- 1 kohlrabi
- 1 piece (approx. 4 cm long) ginger
- 500 g carrots
- 1 can (400 ml) coconut milk
- 500 ml vegetable stock
- 1 tbsp coconut oil
- 1 tbsp turmeric
- 1-2 teaspoons of curry powder
- ½ bunch of parsley
- Salt & pepper

1. Wash and clean the vegetables, peel the potatoes and kohlrabi. Just like the carrots, cut into thin sticks.
2. Peel the ginger thinly and finely chop it.
3. Fry in coconut oil in a tall saucepan while stirring.
4. Add the spices, coconut milk and vegetable stock and simmer covered for 15 minutes.
5. In the meantime, wash the parsley, shake it dry and chop it finely.
6. Put half of the soup in a bowl. Puree the rest in the pot, add the other half again.
7. Bring to the boil again briefly, season with salt and pepper and serve sprinkled with parsley.

Nutritional Value per Serving

331 Kcal	24g Fat	24g Carbs	5g Protein	7g Fiber

Kohlrabi And Chervil Cream Soup

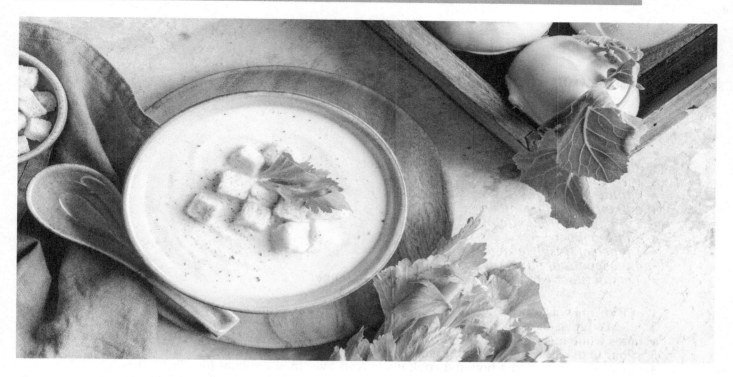

Preparation Time: 20 min

Ingredients for 2 people

- 2 (approx. 600 g) kohlrabi
- 1 onion
- 1 tbsp olive oil
- ½ l vegetable stock
- 300 ml (1.5% fat) milk
- Salt & pepper
- 40 g chervil
- ½ bunch of parsley

1. Halve, clean and peel the kohlrabi. Peel the onion and cut it into large cubes with the kohlrabi.
2. Sauté both in a saucepan in oil over medium heat for 2-3 minutes. P
3. our in the stock and milk, season everything with salt and pepper and bring to a boil once.
4. Cook for about 15 minutes with the lid closed.
5. In the meantime, wash the chervil and parsley, shake dry, pluck some chervil leaves from the stalks, and set them aside.
6. Roughly chop the remaining chervil and parsley with the stems. Add the herbs to the vegetables.
7. Take the pot off the stove and puree everything with a hand blender.
8. Season the soup with salt and pepper.
9. Serve sprinkled with the chervil that you have set aside. In addition, 1 slice of whole meal bread tastes good per serving.

Nutritional Value per Serving

250 Kcal	13 g Fat	19g Carbs	11g Protein	6 g Fiber	21mg Purine	405 mg Calcium

Cauliflower And Fennel Soup With Pumpkin Seeds

Preparation Time: 18 min

Ingredients for 2 people:

- *300 g cauliflower florets*
- *alternatively: Romanesco or broccoli florets*
- *1 (about 150 g) mainly waxy potatoes*
- *2 tablespoons of cold-pressed olive oil*
- *400 ml (1.5% fat) milk*
- *1/4 l gluten-free vegetable stock*
- *Salt & pepper*
- *1 pinch of freshly grated nutmeg*
- *4 teaspoons of pumpkin seeds*
- *1 small tuber (approx. 150 g, with green) of fennel*

1. Clean and wash the cauliflower. Peel the potato and cut it into cubes.
2. Heat 1 tablespoon of oil in a saucepan, sauté cauliflower and potatoes over medium heat for 3-4 minutes while turning.
3. Pour in the milk and stock and season with salt, pepper and nutmeg.
4. Bring everything to a boil and cook uncovered over medium heat for 15-20 minutes, stirring occasionally.
5. In the meantime, coarsely chop the pumpkin seeds (note: if you have ulcerative colitis, diverticulosis and Crohn's disease, grate them finely) and roast them lightly in a pan without fat.
6. Take out and let cool on a plate.
7. Clean and wash the fennel, quarter lengthways, remove the stalk and put the greens aside for garnish. Cut the fennel crosswise into fine strips.
8. Heat the remaining oil in a pan and sauté the fennel over medium heat for 2-3 minutes, keep warm.
9. Finely puree the soup with the hand blender and season with salt, pepper and nutmeg.
10. Distribute on deep plates and place the fennel strips on top.
11. Sprinkle with (ground) pumpkin seeds and garnish with fennel greens.

Nutritional Value per Serving

350 Kcal	18g Fat	28g Carbs	15g Protein	8 g Fiber

Broccoli Cream Soup

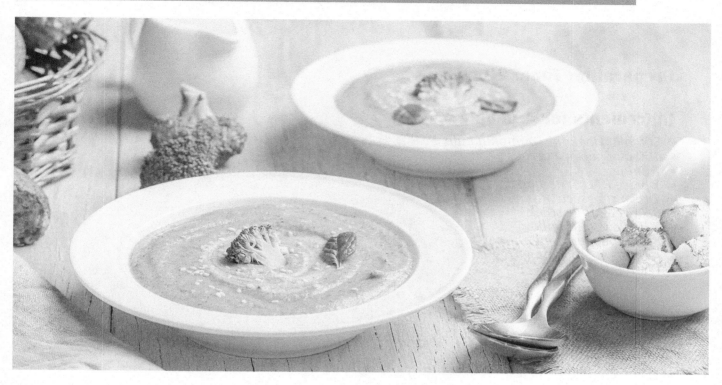

Preparation Time: 15 min

Ingredients for 4 people

- *600 g broccoli*
- *1 tbsp rapeseed oil*
- *1 onion*
- *2 cloves of garlic*
- *750 ml vegetable stock*
- *100 ml reduced-fat cream*
- *parsley*
- *salt & pepper*

1. Clean and roughly cut the broccoli (alternatively: thaw frozen broccoli). Peel and roughly chop the onion and garlic.
2. Heat the oil in a stock pot and sauté broccoli, onion and garlic cubes for five minutes. Pour in the stock and cream and bring to a boil. Cover and simmer for 15 minutes. In the meantime, wash and finely chop the parsley.
3. Puree the soup finely and season with pepper, chopped parsley and a little salt.

Nutritional Value per Serving

110 Kcal	4g Fat	7g Carbs	6g Protein	5g Fiber

Pumpkin Soup With Ginger and Coconut

Preparation Time: 20 min

Ingredients for 4 people

- *500 g of Hokkaido pumpkin pulp*
- *400 g of peeled carrots*
- *1 onion*
- *1 piece (3 cm) of ginger*
- *1 tbsp rapeseed oil*
- *0.7 l vegetable stock*
- *330 g coconut milk*
- *Salt & pepper*
- *Juice of half a lemon*
- *Pumpkin seeds*

1. Dice the pumpkin (preferably with the skin) and carrots.
2. Peel and dice the onion and ginger as well. Braise everything in rapeseed oil.
3. Pour in the broth and cook until soft for about 20 minutes. Then puree very finely.
4. Stir in the coconut milk and season with salt, pepper and lemon juice.
5. Heat again and serve garnished with pumpkin seeds.

Nutritional Value per Serving

266 Kcal	21g Fat	14g Carbs	5g Protein

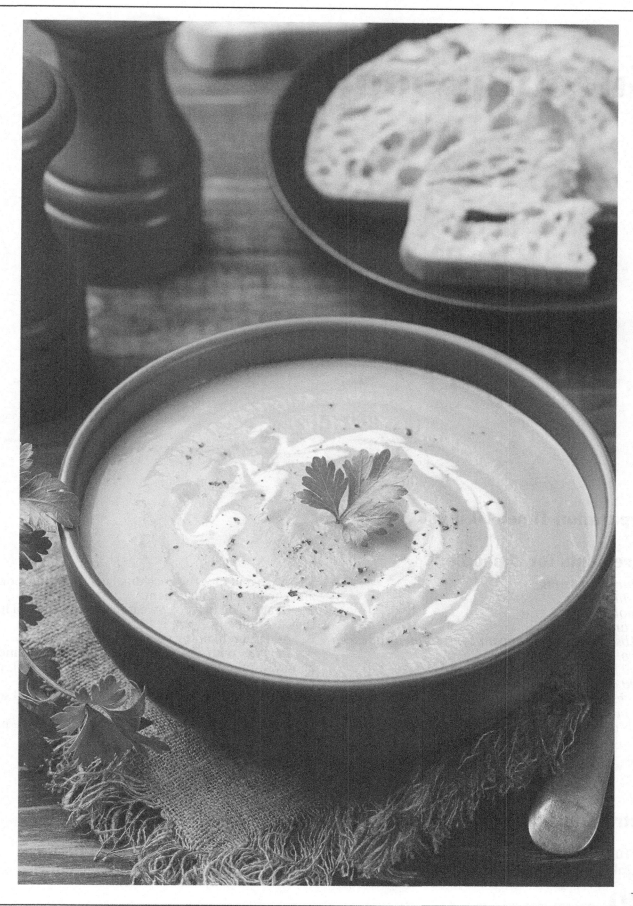

Zucchini Soup

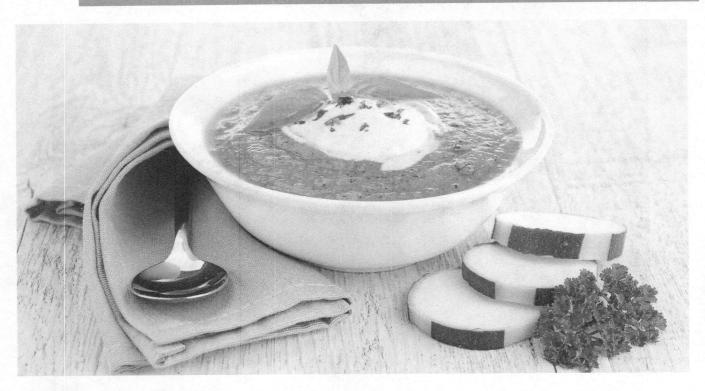

Preparation Time: 10 min

Ingredients for 4 people:

- 2 large zucchinis
- 1 onion
- 2 potatoes
- 2 carrots
- 1 tbsp (sesame oil, coconut fat, refined rapeseed or olive oil) frying oil
- 500 ml vegetable stock
- 100 g (natural, 15% fat in dry matter) cream cheese
- ½ bunch of parsley
- salt and pepper

1. Wash and dice the zucchini. Peel the onion, potatoes and carrots, then dice them.
2. Heat the oil in a pot. Sweat the onion cubes in it until they are golden yellow.
3. Add the remaining vegetables and fry briefly.
4. Deglaze with the vegetable stock and simmer for about 10 minutes. When the vegetables are soft, puree the soup.
5. Stir the cream cheese into the warm soup and season with salt and pepper.
6. Wash and finely chop the parsley and serve on top of the soup.

Nutritional Value per Serving

210 Kcal	16g Fat	7g Carbs	23g Protein	4g Fiber

Snacks

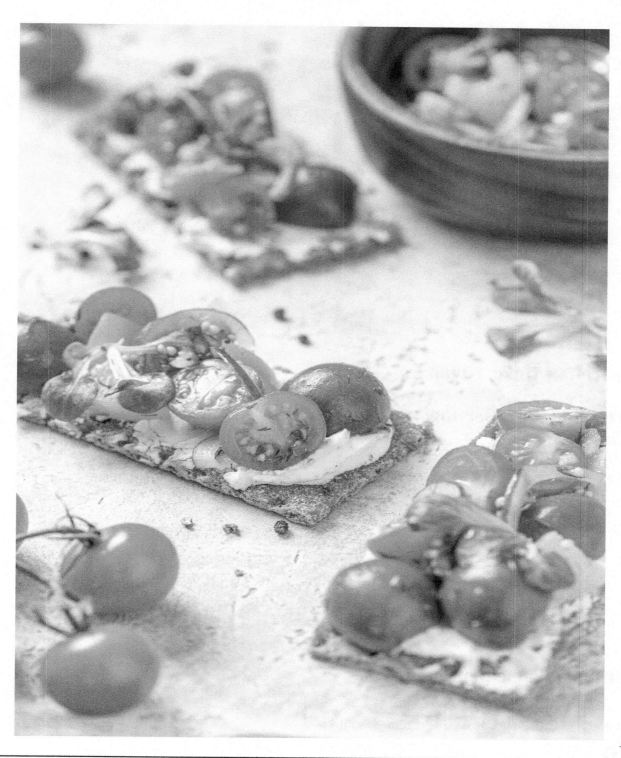

Olive Dip

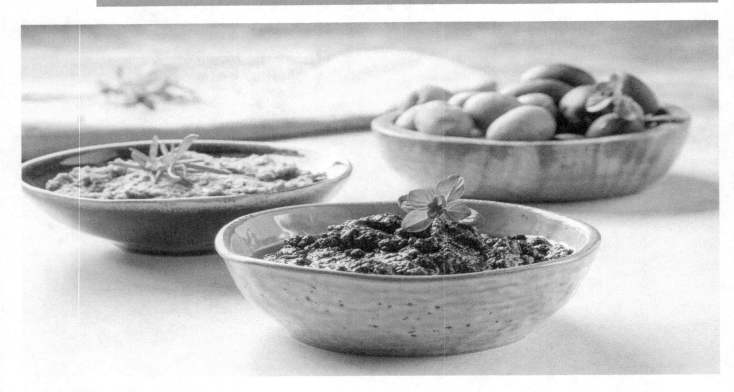

Preparation Time: 10 min

Ingredients for 8 Servings:

- 1 clove of garlic
- 200 g green pitted olives
- 100 g ground almonds
- 2 tbsp chopped parsley
- 70 ml of olive oil
- Salt & pepper

1. Peel the garlic clove and finely chop it together with the olives in a blender or a tall mixing bowl with a hand blender.
2. Add the remaining ingredients and mix everything well.

Nutritional Value per Serving

190 Kcal	19g Fat	2g Carbs	3g Protein	3g Fiber

Mexican Corn Bread with Buttermilk and Lots of Chilies

Preparation Time: 20 min
Ready in 1h 10 min

Ingredients for 16 Discs:

- *2 red chili peppers*
- *6 jalapeños*
- *2 eggs*
- *50 g butter*
- *200 g whole wheat flour*
- *1 packet baking powder*
- *325 g corn grits*
- *500 ml buttermilk*
- *50 g liquid honey*
- *1 tbsp rapeseed oil*
- *salt*

1. Halve the chili peppers lengthways, core, wash and chop.
2. Finely chop the jalapeños. Melt the butter and let it cool down a bit.
3. Sift the flour, baking powder and 1 teaspoon salt into a bowl and mix with the corn grits.
4. Mix the buttermilk, honey, eggs and melted butter together.
5. Add to the flour together with the chilies and jalapeños and stir everything into a smooth batter.
6. Brush a 30 cm long loaf pan with oil and pour in the dough. Bake in the preheated oven on the 2nd shelf from the bottom on an oven rack at 180 ° C (air circulation: 160 ° C, gas: level 2–3) for 35–40 minutes.
7. Let the cornbread cool in the tin for 10 minutes, then turn it out onto an oven rack and let it cool completely.
8. Corn bread tastes simply coated with butter but is also a good accompaniment to chilies and stews.

Nutritional Value per Serving

169 Kcal	5g Fat	26g Carbs	5g Protein	2.4 g Fiber	2.3g Added Sugar

Spelt and Quark Rolls With Apple

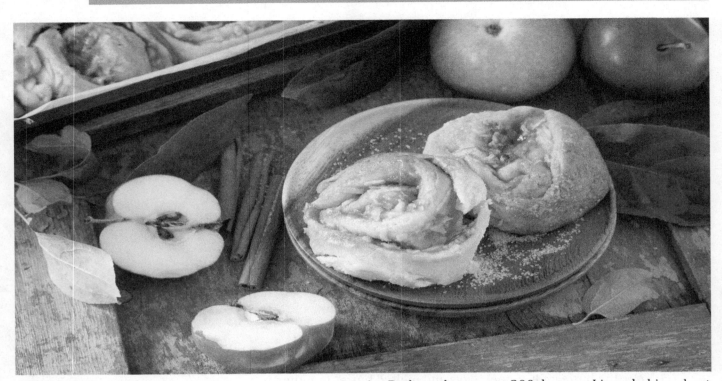

Preparation Time: 20 min

Ingredients for 8 pieces:

- 250 g low-fat quark
- 1 (size M) egg
- 2 tbsp walnut oil
- salt
- 250 g wholegrain spelt flour
- 50 g of oat bran
- 1 packet of tartar baking powder
- ½ teaspoon cinnamon powder
- ½ (approx. 100 g, e.g., Elstar) apple
- some spelt flour

1. Preheat the oven to 200 degrees. Line a baking sheet with parchment paper.
2. Mix the quark and egg with the oil and a pinch of salt in a mixing bowl with a whisk until smooth.
3. Mix the flour with the oat bran, baking powder and cinnamon in a second bowl. Quarter, peel and core the apple.
4. Grate coarsely on the vegetable grater and stir immediately into the flour mixture. Add to the quark mixture and knead everything into a smooth dough using the dough hook of the hand mixer.
5. Shape the dough into a roll with your hands on the lightly floured work surface and cut it into 8 pieces. Shape each piece of dough into a ball between the palms of your hands and place on the baking sheet.
6. Cut the rolls crosswise about 1 cm deep with a sharp knife and bake in the oven in the lower third for about 20 minutes.
7. Take out, let cool down briefly and serve lukewarm or cold.
8. Top with savory or sweet as desired.

Tip: *The rolls keep for up to 3 days. You can also freeze them well, defrost them again if necessary and toast them briefly.*

Nutritional Value per Piece

210 Kcal	5g Fat	28g Carbs	10g Protein	4g Fiber

Energy Balls

Preparation Time: 60 min

Ingredients for approx 20 pieces:

- *1 tbsp lime juice*
- *alternatively: 1 tbsp water*
- *50 g (small leaf/tender) oat flakes*
- *75 g dried (without stone) dates*
- *50 g desiccated coconut*
- *2 tbsp ground sesame seeds*

1. Mix the oatmeal with the lime juice in a bowl.
2. Finely chop the dried fruit together with the desiccated coconut in a lightning chopper, adding a little water or lime juice if necessary.
3. Knead the mixture with the oat flakes, form about 20 balls of the same size (diameter approx. 2 cm) and roll them one after the other in the ground sesame seeds.
4. Line a baking sheet with parchment paper, distribute the balls on it and leave to dry for at least 1 hour.
5. Store in the refrigerator.

Nutritional Value per Piece

42 Kcal	2g Fat	4g Carbs	1g Protein	1 g Fiber

Millet Pancakes

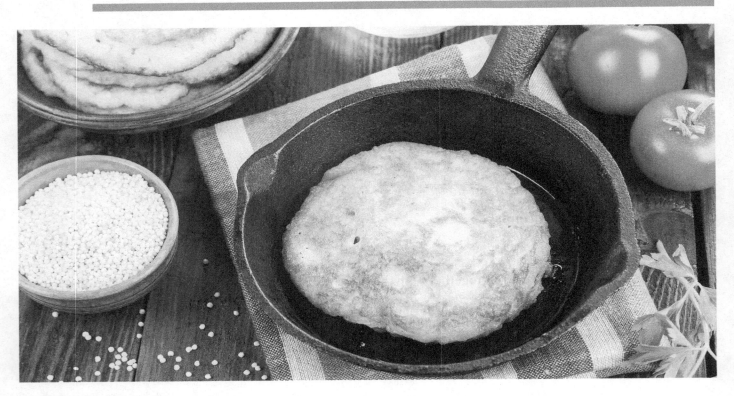

Preparation Time: 60 min

Ingredients for 4 people

- 1 medium-sized carrot
- 250 g millet
- 1 onion
- 2 tbsp soy flour
- 50 g sunflower seeds
- 50 g sesame seeds
- salt
- olive oil

1. Clean and finely dice the carrot.
2. Meanwhile, bring about 650 ml of water with about 1/2 teaspoon of salt to the boil.
3. Simmer the millet with the diced carrot for about 30 minutes and then let it soak for another 5 minutes.
4. In the meantime, cut the onion into small cubes.
5. Put the cooked millet and carrot mash in a bowl.
6. Add soy flour, coarsely chopped sunflower seeds, sesame seeds and onion cubes and mix everything together well.
7. Shape the millet dough into flat buffers with moistened hands.
8. Gently fry them little by little in a little olive oil.

Nutritional Value per Serving

425 Kcal	18g Fat	51g Carbs	15g Protein	6g Fiber

Fried Mini Peppers in Olive Oil

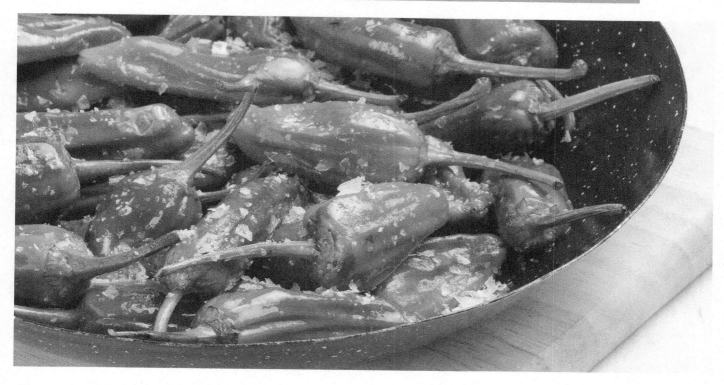

Preparation Time: 10 min

Ingredients for 2 people:

- *300 g small green pepper (preferably pimientos de padrón)*
- *2 tbsp olive oil*
- *coarse sea salt*
- *pepper*

1. Wash the peppers and dry them thoroughly with kitchen paper.
2. Heat the olive oil in a large non-stick pan.
3. Add peppers and fry for 4-5 minutes over high heat, stirring constantly.
4. Season the paprika with coarse sea salt and pepper.

Nutritional Value per Serving

115 Kcal	10g Fat	4g Carbs	1g Protein	5g Fiber	0g Added Sugar

Avocado Feta Dip

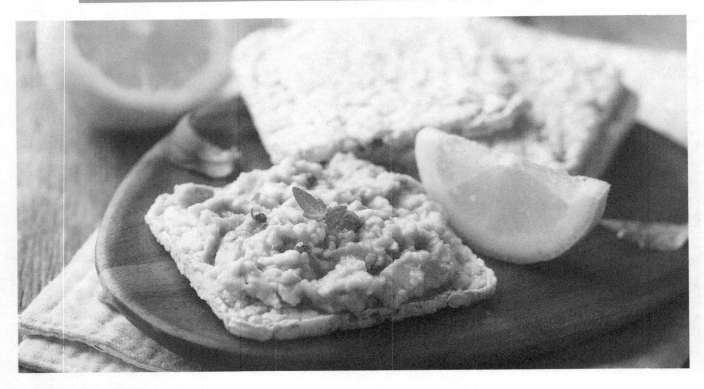

Preparation Time: 10 min

Ingredients for 1 person:

- 1 avocado
- 1 toe garlic
- 35 g Feta
- 1 lime
- salt
- pepper

1. Halve the avocado, remove the core and peel.
2. Put the pulp in a bowl, and squeeze the lime.
3. Peel and finely chop the clove of garlic, add to the avocado with feta and lime juice.
4. Mash everything with a fork to a creamy mass.
5. Season to taste with salt and pepper.

Nutritional Value per Serving

290 Kcal	22 g Fat	13g Carbs	7g Protein	4 g Fiber

Banana bread

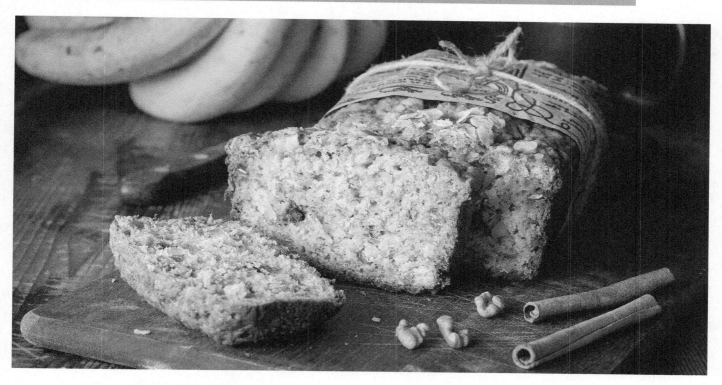

Preparation Time: 50 min

Ingredients for 1 bread:

- *3 ripe bananas*
- *3 eggs*
- *50 g ground almonds*
- *100 g spelt flour*
- *100 g of oat flour*
- *alternatively: 100 g oat flakes*
- *1 teaspoon vanilla powder*
- *1 tbsp brown cane sugar*
- *2 tbsp coconut oil*
- *1 teaspoon Baking powder*
- *1 teaspoon cinnamon*
- *1 pinch of coarse sea salt*

1. Preheat the oven to 170 degrees circulating air.
2. Peel the bananas, break them roughly and whisk well with the eggs, vanilla, sugar and fat in a mixing bowl.
3. Mix in the almonds, spelt and oat flour, salt, baking powder and cinnamon and mix everything into a batter. Its consistency is right when it falls from the spoon with a tough tear.
4. Spread the dough out in a loaf pan and place it in the oven. Bake for 30-35 minutes until the desired degree of browning is achieved. Possibly check whether the cake is done by piercing it with a wooden stick.
5. Take out of the oven and let cool down briefly in the tin.
6. After 15 minutes, turn over and let cool down further.

Nutritional Value per Serving per Slice of approx 55 grams

88 Kcal	4g Fat	10g Carbs	3g Protein	1g Fiber

Salmon and Spinach Roll

Preparation Time: 60 min

Ingredients per 4 people

- *125 g frozen spinach*
- *4 eggs*
- *50 g (max. 30 fat in dry matter) grated cheese*
- *250 g smoked salmon*
- *200 g (max. 16% fat) herbal cream cheese*
- *Salt & pepper*
- *1 lemon*
- *some grated parmesan*

1. Thaw the spinach and squeeze it out well.
2. Beat the eggs until frothy.
3. Mix the spinach, salt, pepper and grated cheese with the egg mixture.
4. Line a baking sheet with baking paper and sprinkle with parmesan; spread the spinach mixture on top. Bake for 10 minutes at 200 degrees and let it cool down. Then turn it over so that the filling comes on the cheese side.
5. Brush with herbal cream cheese spread the salmon on top and drizzle with the lemon juice.
6. Roll up the whole thing tightly, wrap in cling film and refrigerate for at least 6 hours.
7. Then cut into slices of any thickness.

Nutritional Value per Serving

347 Kcal	22g Fat	3g Carbs	32g Protein	1g Fiber

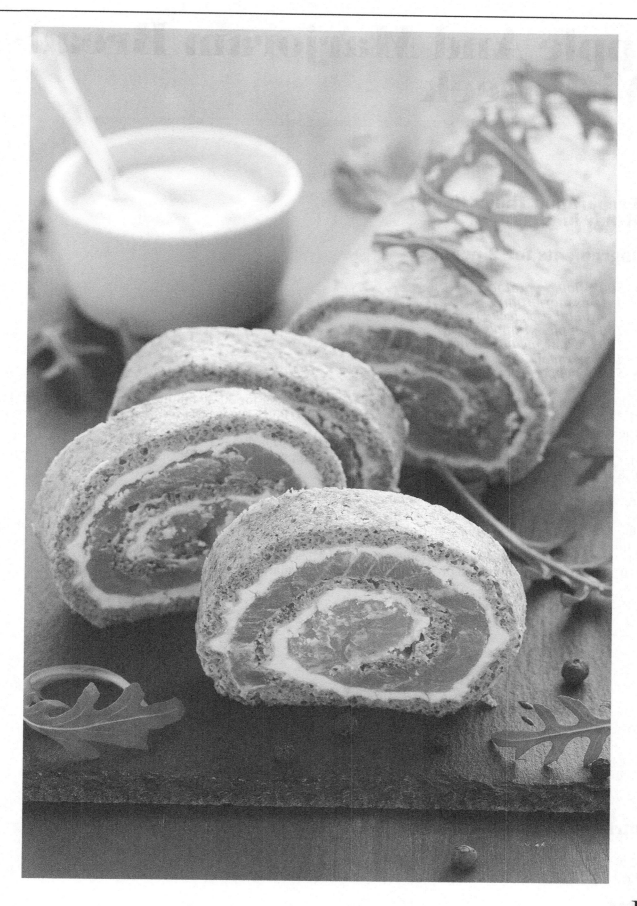

Apple And Marjoram Breads With Leek

Preparation Time: 30 min
Ready in 1h

Ingredients for 2 people:

- 300 g floury potatoes
- 4 stems marjoram
- 70 g small stick leek (1 small stick leek)
- 150 g apples (1 apple)
- 100 g whole meal spelt bread (2 slices)
- 1 tsp germ oil
- Salt & pepper

1. Wash the potatoes and cook with the skin in boiling water for 20-30 minutes, depending on their size.
2. In the meantime, rinse the marjoram and shake dry. Pluck the leaves, set some aside and finely chop the rest.
3. Halve the leek lengthways, wash, clean and cut into strips about 1 cm wide (only the light).
4. Wash the apple, rub dry and cut all around into approx. 1 cm thick slices from the core. Finely dice the apple slices.
5. Heat the oil in a coated pan.
6. Add the leek and cook covered for about 6 minutes over low heat.
7. Add the apple cubes and chopped marjoram and sauté for 1 minute. Season with salt and pepper.
8. Drain the potatoes, rinse under cold water, peel and press through a potato press into a bowl while still warm.
9. Stir in the apple and leek vegetables, season with salt, pepper and leave to cool.
10. Spread the spread on the bread slices, garnish with marjoram leaves and serve.

Nutritional Value per Serving

229 Kcal	2g Fat	44g Carbs	6g Protein	9g Fiber	0g Added Sugar

Avocado Crostini With Goat Cheese and Cherry Tomatoes

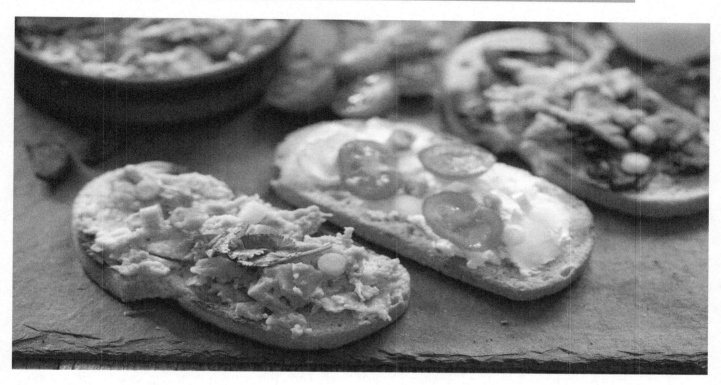

Preparation Time: 35 min

Ingredients for 4 people:

- 200 g ciabatta (1 ciabatta)
- 1 avocado
- ½ lemon
- 1 clove of garlic
- 125 g young goat cheese without rind
- 10 cherry tomatoes z. b. colorful
- ½ fret chives
- Salt & pepper

1. Cut the ciabatta bread into about 1 cm thick slices, spread on the oven rack, bake in a preheated oven at 200 ° C (fan oven 180 ° C, gas: level 3) until golden, remove and let cool slightly.
2. Halve the avocado and remove the stone.
3. Remove the pulp from the skin and place it in a bowl.
4. Squeeze the lemon. Peel and roughly chop the garlic.
5. Coarsely crumble the goat cheese.
6. Add the cheese, 2 teaspoons of lemon juice and garlic to the avocado.
7. Puree everything finely, season with salt, pepper and possibly a little lemon juice.
8. Wash, drain and quarter tomatoes.
9. Spread the avocado cream on the ciabatta slices and top with pieces of tomato.
10. Rinse the chives, shake dry, cut the stalks once or twice and spread on the crostini. Serve immediately.

Nutritional Value per Serving

307 Kcal	18g Fat	27g Carbs	8g Protein	3g Fiber	0g Added Sugar

Tuna Muffins

Preparation Time: 30 min

Ingredients for 12 Muffins:

- *2 cans (in its own juice) of tuna*
- *100 g Gouda*
- *300 g pumpkin meat*
- *1 red pepper*
- *1 large onion*
- *2 tbsp chopped (fresh or frozen) dill*
- *4 eggs*
- *2 tbsp reduced-fat cream cheese*
- *Salt & pepper*
- *noble sweet paprika powder*

1. Preheat the oven to 200 degrees.
2. Grease a muffin tin with a bit of oil using a brush.
3. Drain the tuna and grate the cheese.
4. Chop the pumpkin flesh (e.g., Hokkaido) very finely (possibly with a lightning chopper or a food processor).
5. Wash the peppers and remove the seeds. As well as chop the onion very finely.
6. Put all ingredients in a mixing bowl and mix thoroughly with a mixer.
7. Season to taste with the spices.
8. Spread the mixture on the muffin tin and bake in the oven for about 30 minutes.

Nutritional Value per Muffin

92.8 Kcal	5g Fat	3g Carbs	10.1g Protein	1g Fiber

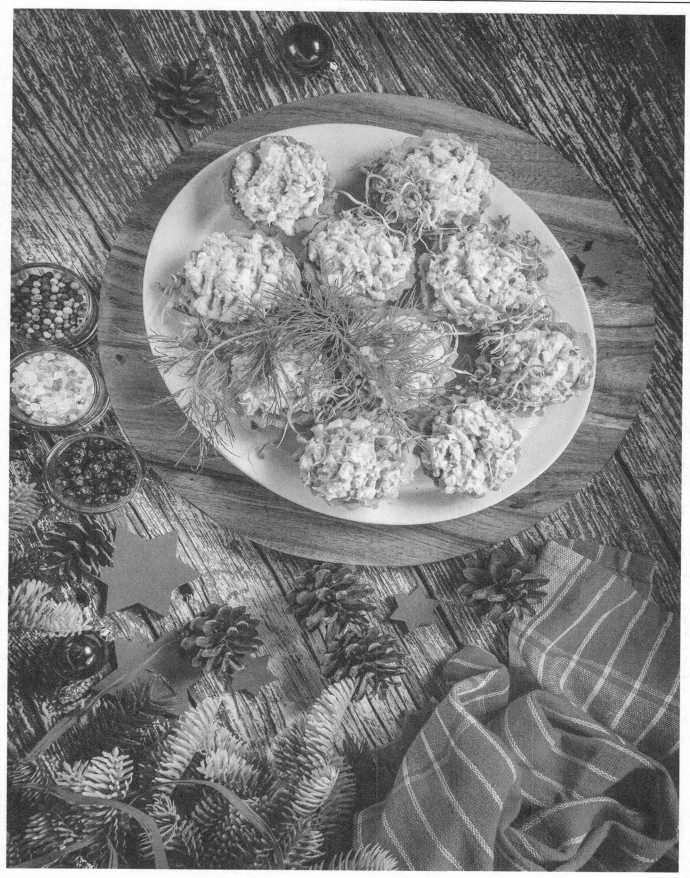

Vegan Banana Bread

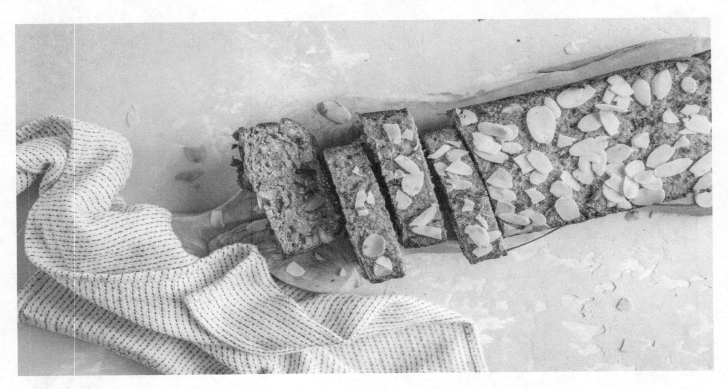

Preparation Time: 35 min

Ingredients for a loaf Pan (16 slices)

- *3 ripe bananas*
- *90 ml neutral (e.g., coconut oil) oil*
- *100 ml (e.g., oat drink) plant drink*
- *1 pack of vanilla sugar*
- *50 g ground almonds*
- *190 g whole meal spelt flour*
- *1 tbsp starch*
- *1 pinch of sea salt*
- *1 teaspoon baking soda*
- *alternatively: tartar baking powder*
- *if you like: 1 pinch of cinnamon*

1. Preheat the oven to 170 degrees circulating air.
2. Peel and roughly chop the bananas. Place in a mixing bowl with the oil, vegetable drink and sugar and whisk with the mixer.
3. Add dry ingredients and work everything into a smooth batter.
4. Put the dough in a greased and lightly floured loaf pan.
5. Bake for about 35 minutes. After 30 minutes, make a cooking test with a wooden stick, possibly switch off the oven.
6. After removing the cake, use a knife to loosen the sides from the pan. Do not fall out of the mold until it has cooled down.

Nutritional Value per Slice(with 16 slices)

131 Kcal	8g Fat	13g Carbs	3g Protein	2g Fiber	1 BE

Desserts

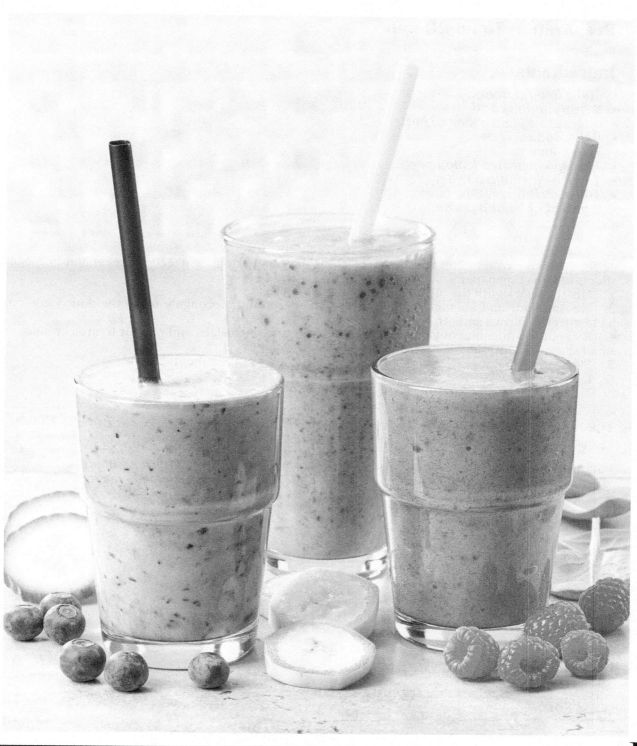

Cookies Made From Curd and Oil Dough

Preparation Time: 20 min

Ingredients:

- 200 g low-fat quark
- 8 tbsp sunflower oil
- alternatively: 80 g melted butter
- 8 tbsp milk
- 75 g honey
- 1 teaspoon grated lemon peel
- 1 pinch of vanilla powder
- 400 g spelt flour (type 630)
- 1 packet of baking powder

1. Preheat the oven to 200 degrees circulating air (top/bottom heat 220 degrees) and line 2 baking sheets with baking paper.
2. Mix the quark with the oil, milk, honey and lemon zest.
3. Mix the flour and baking powder and knead everything thoroughly using the dough hook of the hand mixer to form a smooth dough.
4. Roll out the dough about 5 mm high on a floured work surface and cut out figures or smooth out small shapes as desired.
5. Place on the baking sheet and bake in the preheated oven for about 7 minutes.
6. Let cool on a wire rack.

Tip: *It is best to enjoy the pastries fresh. It can be kept airtight for 1-2 days, but can also be frozen for longer storage times. Thaw in portions at room temperature.*

Variant:Before *baking, brush the biscuits with 1 whisked egg yolk and sprinkle lightly with sugar or granulated sugar. However, it is better to omit this decoration in the case of inflammatory diseases.*

Nutritional Value per Serving

320 Kcal	1g Fat	4g Carbs	1g Protein	0.2 g Fiber

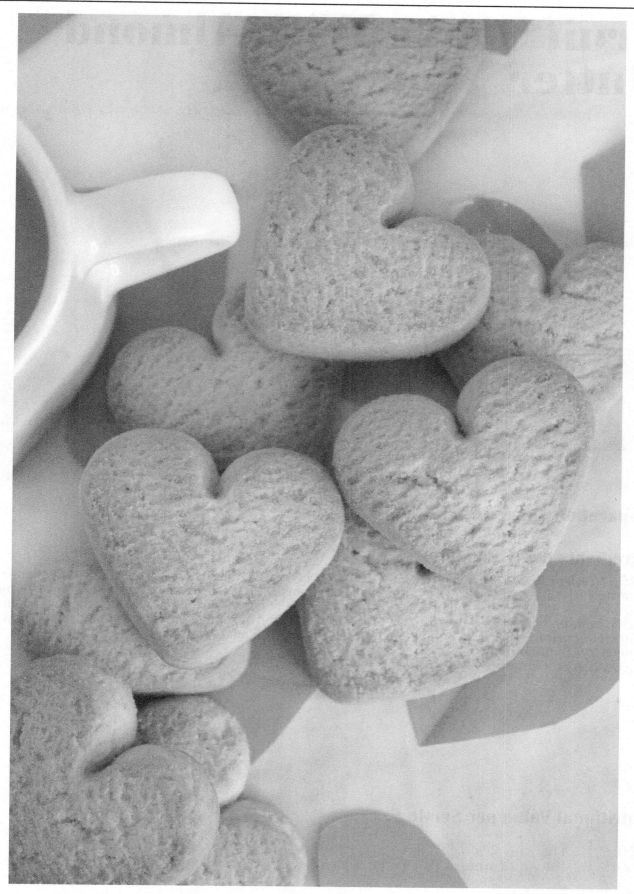

Fruit Shake With Almond Butter

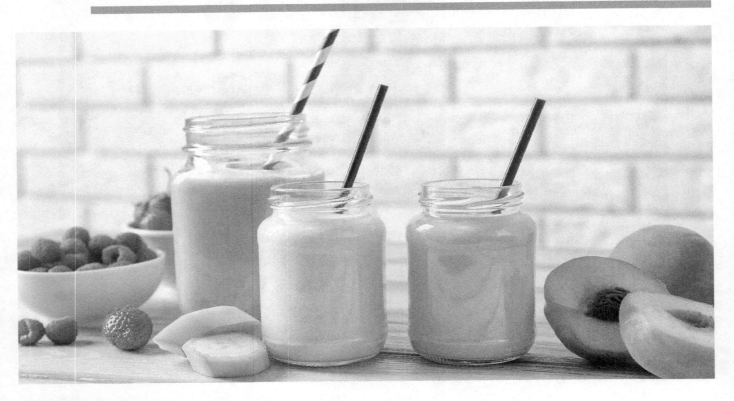

Preparation Time: 10 min

Ingredients per 1 people

- 125 g (fresh or frozen) raspberries
- alternatively: 1 peach or 125 g (without skin) melon
- 1 tbsp almond butter
- 150 ml oat drink
- 1 pinch of cinnamon
- 1 teaspoon maple syrup

1. Wash or defrost the raspberries (or wash the peach, roughly cut it and remove the stone or core of the melon).
2. Put the fruit together with the other ingredients in a powerful mixer or whisk well in a high mixing bowl with a hand blender.

Nutritional Value per Serving

218 Kcal	11g Fat	20g Carbs	8g Protein	9g Fiber

Smoothie with Avocado and Pears

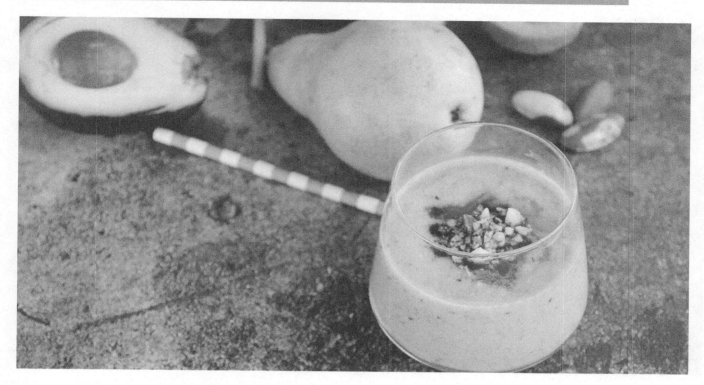

Preparation Time: 10 min

Ingredients per 1 Serving:

- ½ avocado
- 1-2 pears
- 1 squeezed orange
- 50 g baby spinach or lamb's lettuce
- as desired: lemon juice
- 1 tbsp linseed oil

1. Peel the avocado and fruit, remove the stones and roughly chop the pulp.
2. Wash the green leaves thoroughly.
3. Puree all ingredients well in a blender or with a hand blender.

Nutritional Value per Serving

180 Kcal	10g Fat	19g Carbs	2g Protein	5g Fiber

Smoothie With Raspberries, Peach And Lettuce

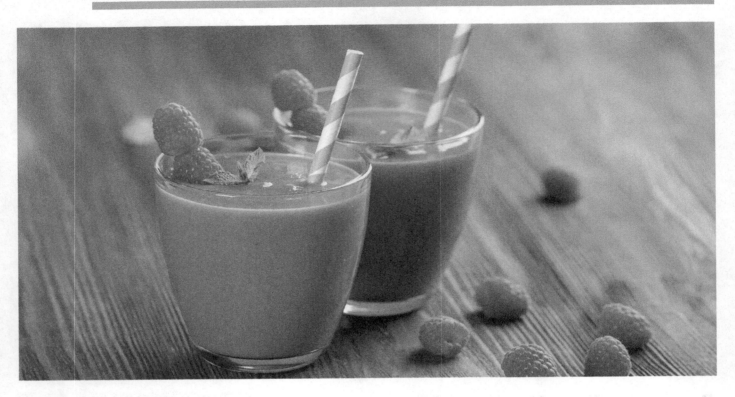

Preparation Time: 10 min

Ingredients for 1 Serving:

- 150 ml of water
- 50 g raspberries
- 5-6 leaves of lettuce
- 1 peach
- 1 tbsp linseed oil

1. Rinse the fruit and lettuce, remove the stone from the peach and chop the pulp.
2. Puree all ingredients together in a blender or with a hand blender.

Nutritional Value per Serving

100 Kcal	6g Fat	8g Carbs	2g Protein	4g Fiber

Chocolate Strawberries With Cardamom

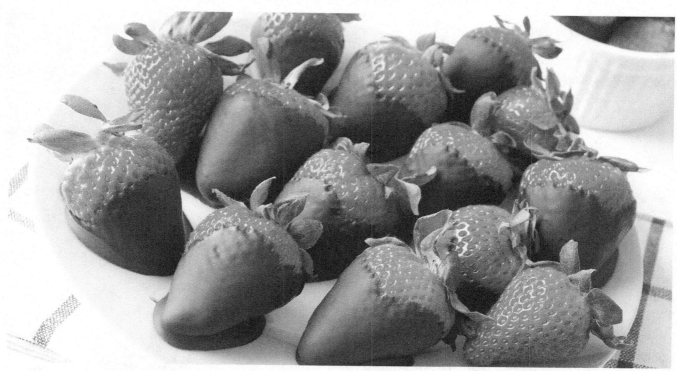

Preparation Time: 20 min
Ready in 30 min

Ingredients for 4 people:

- *400 g strawberries*
- *2 cardamom pods*
- *100 g dark chocolate couverture (at least 72% cocoa)*

1. Put the strawberries in a colander, wash carefully and pat dry.
2. Break open the cardamom pods and remove the seeds. Finely crush the cardamom seeds in a mortar.
3. Roughly chop the couverture and place in a small beater.
4. Add the cardamom.
5. Melt the couverture in a hot water bath while stirring.
6. Take hold of the strawberries by the stem and dip 2/3 of the way into the liquid couverture.
7. Place the chocolate strawberries on baking paper and let the couverture dry.
8. Chill the chocolate strawberries until ready to serve.

Nutritional Value per Serving

156 Kcal	8g Fat	17g Carbs	3g Protein	4.4g Fiber	0g dded Sugar

Smoothie with Mango, Banana and Carrot Greens

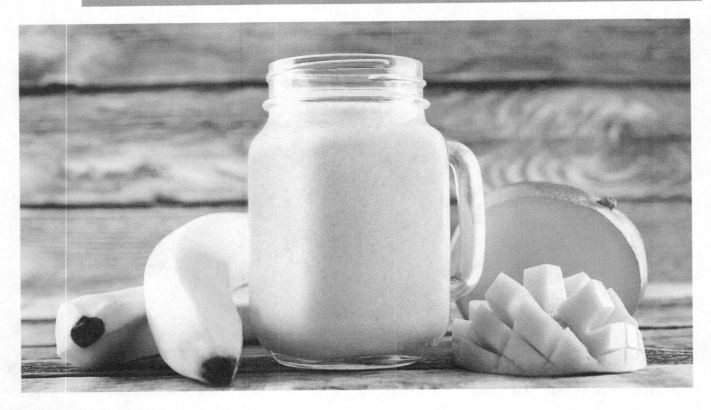

Preparation Time: 15 min

Ingredients for 2 servings:

- 400 ml of water
- 150 g baby spinach or romaine lettuce
- Green from 3 carrots
- 1 orange
- 1 mango
- 1 banana
- 1 tbsp linseed oil

1. Preparation time: 15 mins
2. Preparation steps
3. Peel and roughly chop the fruit, loosening the mango meat from the core.
4. Wash the lettuce and carrot leaves well.
5. Finely puree all ingredients together in a blender or with a hand blender.
6. Leftovers from the smoothie can be kept in the refrigerator for half a day (shake well before drinking).

Nutritional Value per Serving

180 Kcal	7g Fat	22g Carbs	4g Protein	5 g Fiber

Smoothie With Spinach And Strawberries

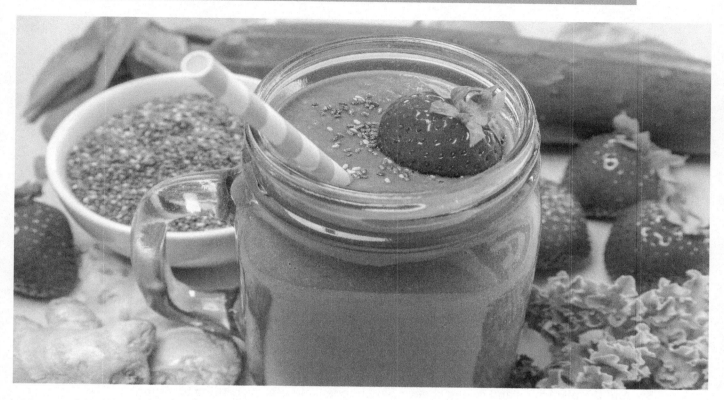

Preparation Time: 10 min

Ingredients for 2 people:

- *150 ml of water*
- *250 g spinach*
- *5 large strawberries*
- *1 pear*
- *1 tbsp linseed oil*
- *1 tbsp wheat germ oil*

1. Wash and clean the strawberries.
2. Wash the pear, quarter it and remove the core.
3. Wash the fresh spinach. Frozen spinach is also suitable - if necessary, roughly chop.
4. Finely puree all ingredients together in a blender or with a hand blender.

Nutritional Value per Serving

130 Kcal	7g Fat	11g Carbs	4g Protein	5g Fiber

Baked Figs With Cream Cheese And Pistachio Filling

Preparation Time: 25 min

Ingredients for 2 people:

- 20 g pistachio kernels (1 heaped tablespoon)
- 2 stems basil
- 6 fresh, ripe figs
- 100 g grainy cream cheese (13% fat)
- Salt & pepper
- 1 small head romaine lettuce
- 1 tbsp white wine vinegar
- 2 ½ tbsp olive oil

1. Roughly chop the pistachio nuts and lightly toast them in a pan without fat.
2. Wash the basil, shake dry and chop the leaves. Put in a bowl.
3. Wash the figs thoroughly, pat dry and cut off a lid each time.
4. Remove the pulp with a teaspoon and add to the bowl.
5. Add the pistachios and cream cheese. Salt, pepper, and mix everything together.
6. Put the filling in the figs, put the lid back on and place the fruits in the baking dish. Bake in a preheated oven at 200 ° C (fan oven: 180 ° C, gas: level 2–3) for 12 minutes.
7. Clean, wash, spin dry the lettuce and, if necessary, pluck it into small pieces.
8. Mix a sauce (vinaigrette) from vinegar, oil, salt and pepper and mix with the salad.
9. Place on a platter, place the figs on top and serve.

Nutritional Value per Serving

352 Kcal	18g Fat	33g Carbs	11g Protein	7g Fiber	0g Added Fiber

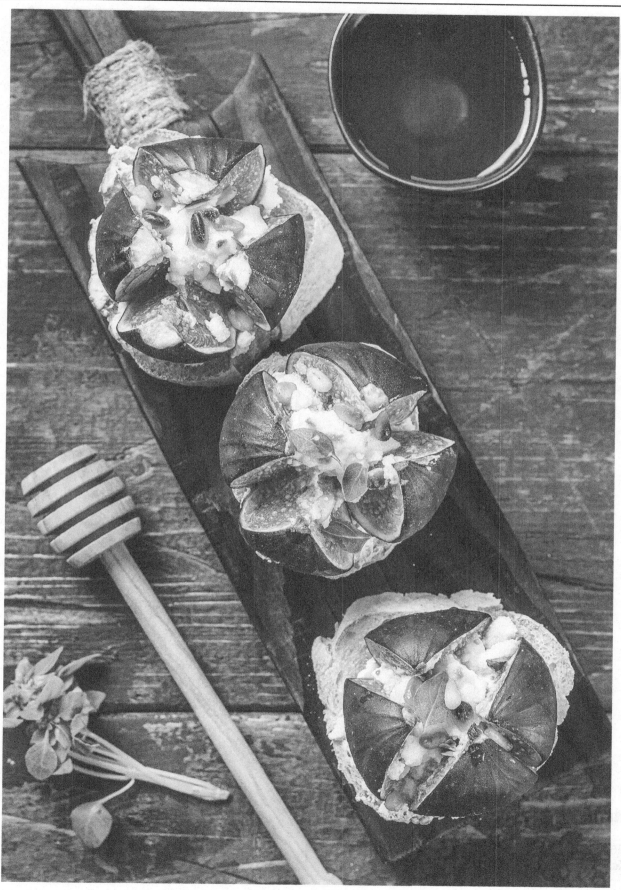

Spicy Melon Cold Peel With Spring Onions

Preparation Time: 1 min

Ingredients for 2 people:

- 750 g watermelon (0.5 watermelons; well chilled)
- 4 branches lemon thyme
- 200 ml classic vegetable broth
- Salt & pepper
- 3 spring onions
- 1 tbsp apple syrup

1. Cut the watermelon into wedges with a large knife and peel it.
2. Core the melon wedges and cut them into pieces.
3. Wash the thyme and shake dry. Strip the leaves from 2 branches, finely puree with melon and stock in a blender or hand blender. Salt and pepper.
4. Wash the spring onions, drain, clean and cut diagonally into rings. Briefly toast in a non-stick frying pan.
5. Add apple syrup, bring to a boil and then let cool down a little.
6. Sprinkle the melon puree with the spring onions, garnish with the remaining thyme and serve.

Nutritional Value per Serving

96 Kcal	0g Fat	20g Carbs	2g Protein	1.5g Fiber	3g Added Sugar

Strawberry Papaya Drink With Kiwi Puree

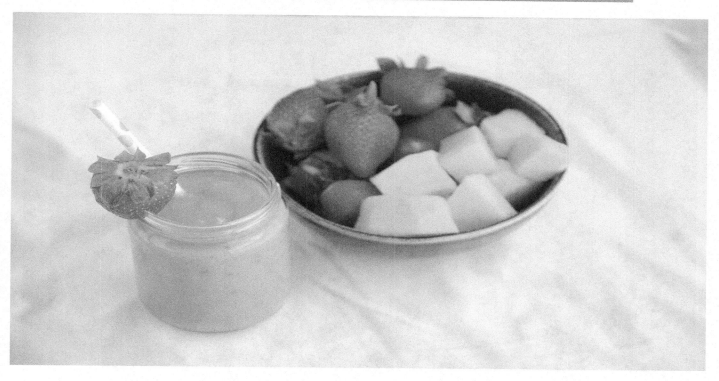

Preparation Time: 10 min

Ingredients for 2 people:

- *2 stems mint*
- *250 g strawberries*
- *2 kiwi fruit*
- *400 g papaya (1 papaya)*

1. Wash the mint, shake dry, pluck the leaves off and set aside.
2. Carefully wash the strawberries, drain them on kitchen paper, clean, roughly chop and place in a tall container. Purée finely with a hand blender and pour into 2 glasses.
3. Peel, halve and dice the kiwi fruit and place it in a tall container.
4. Puree with a hand blender and carefully pour onto the strawberry puree with a spoon.
5. Halve the papaya and remove the seeds with a spoon.
6. Remove the pulp from the skin, roughly chop and also puree with a hand blender.
7. Carefully pour into glasses, garnish with mint and serve immediately.

Nutritional Value per Serving

110 Kcal	1g Fat	20g Carbs	3g Protein	8.5g Fiber	0g Added Sugar

Pineapple And Cucumber Salsa With Spring Onions

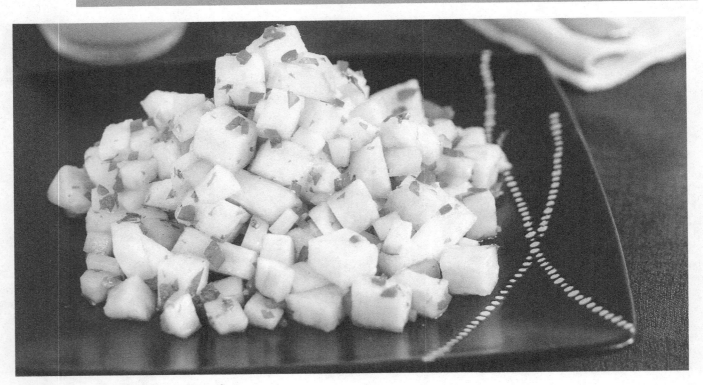

Preparation Time: 15 min
Ready in 45 min

Ingredients for 4 people

- *1 fresh pineapple*
- *250 g cucumber (0.5 cucumber)*
- *1 bunch spring onions*
- *1 small chili pepper*
- *3 tbsp apple cider vinegar*
- *1 tbsp honey*
- *salt*

1. Preparation steps
2. Peel the pineapple. Weigh out 400 g of pulp, dice finely and place in a bowl.
3. Peel the cucumber, cut in half lengthways and core with a spoon. Also, finely dice and mix with the pineapple cubes.
4. Clean and wash the spring onions and cut them into thin rings. Mix in as well.
5. Wash, halve, core and finely chop the chili pepper.
6. Mix with vinegar, honey and a little salt in a small bowl.
7. Pour the sauce over the pineapple and cucumber mixture and fold in.
8. Let steep for 30 minutes, then season to taste again.

Nutritional Value per Serving

91 Kcal	0g Fat	20g Carbs	1g Protein	2.5g Fiber	3g Added Sugar

Chocolate Slices With Raspberries

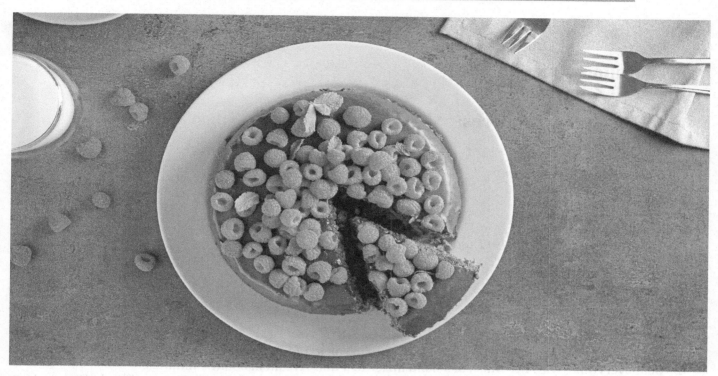

Preparation Time: 30 min
Ready in 3h 10 min

Ingredients for 6 pieces:

- *400 g raspberries*
- *4 eggs*
- *100 g cane sugar plus 2 tablespoons of sugar for the topping*
- *75 g flour*
- *25 g cocoa powder*
- *75 ml orange juice (freshly squeezed at will)*
- *2 tbsp orange liqueur (or 2 tbsp orange juice)*
- *5 tbsp raspberry jelly*
- *250 ml red grape juice*
- *1 packet red cake topping*
- *salt*

1. Separate eggs. Beat the egg whites and a pinch of salt with the hand mixer whisk.
2. Beat egg yolks with 100 g sugar and 2 tablespoons hot water until very creamy.
3. Mix the flour and cocoa and sift. Alternately fold the egg whites and flour mixture into the egg yolk mixture.
4. Cover a baking sheet (30 x 40 cm) with baking paper. Spread the dough on the paper. Bake in the preheated oven at 200 ° C (convection 180 ° C, gas: level 3) on the 2nd rack from the bottom for 12 minutes. Turn the dough to cool on an oven rack.
5. Peel off the baking paper. Mix the orange juice with the liqueur and drizzle over the cake. Cut the cake lengthways into 3 strips.
6. Rinse the raspberries, drain them in a colander and sort.
7. Heat the jelly and brush the surface of the cake strips with it.
8. Lay strips on top of each other. Put the raspberries on top.
9. Prepare the grape juice, remaining sugar and icing according to the packet's instructions and drizzle over the raspberries.
10. Chill for 2 hours. Then cut the cake into pieces.

Nutritional Value per Serving

3335 Kcal	6g Fat	59g Carbs	8g Protein	6.5g Fiber	22g Added Sugar

Strawberry Cake With Lime Icing And Buttermilk Cream

Preparation Time: 35 min
Ready in 2 h

Ingredients for 12 pieces:

- 650 g strawberries
- 2 eggs
- 90 g coconut blossom sugar
- 100 g spelt flour type 630
- 230 ml clear apple juice
- 125 ml whipped cream
- 1 tsp baking powder
- 7 g ground almond kernels (1 teaspoon)
- 1 lime
- 1 packet clear cake topping
- 1 pinch salt
- 4 tbsp buttermilk

1. Put the eggs, 1 pinch of salt, 60 g coconut blossom sugar and 2 tablespoons of hot water in a mixing bowl.
2. Beat everything with the whisk of a hand mixer to a thick cream in about 4 minutes.
3. Mix the flour and baking powder and fold into the cream in 2 portions, one after another, with a whisk.
4. Line the bottom of a springform pan (Ø 24 cm) with baking paper. Pour in the dough, smooth it out and sprinkle with the ground almonds. Bake in the preheated oven at 180 ° C (fan oven 160 ° C, gas: level 2–3) on the middle shelf for 12–15 minutes.
5. Take the tin out of the oven, place it on a wire rack and let it cool down for 5–6 minutes. Then remove the biscuit from the mold and let it cool completely.
6. In the meantime, carefully wash the strawberries in a bowl with cold water, remove them and drain them on kitchen paper. Then clean and cut in half.
7. Place the cooled sponge cake with the almond side up on a cake plate and spread the strawberries on top.
8. Wash the lime with hot water and rub dry. Finely grate the lime peel, halve the lime and squeeze out.
9. Mix the cake icing powder and the remaining coconut blossom sugar in a small saucepan.
10. Gradually stir in the lime zest, apple juice and 2 tablespoons of lime juice and bring everything to a boil while stirring.
11. Spread the icing over the strawberries from the center outwards with a spoon.
12. Chill the cake for at least 20 minutes.
13. Just before serving, whip the cream until stiff and stir in the buttermilk. Serve the cream with the cake.

Nutritional Value for Serving

143 Kcal	5g Fat	20g Carbs	3g Protein	1.5g Fiber	8g Added Sugar

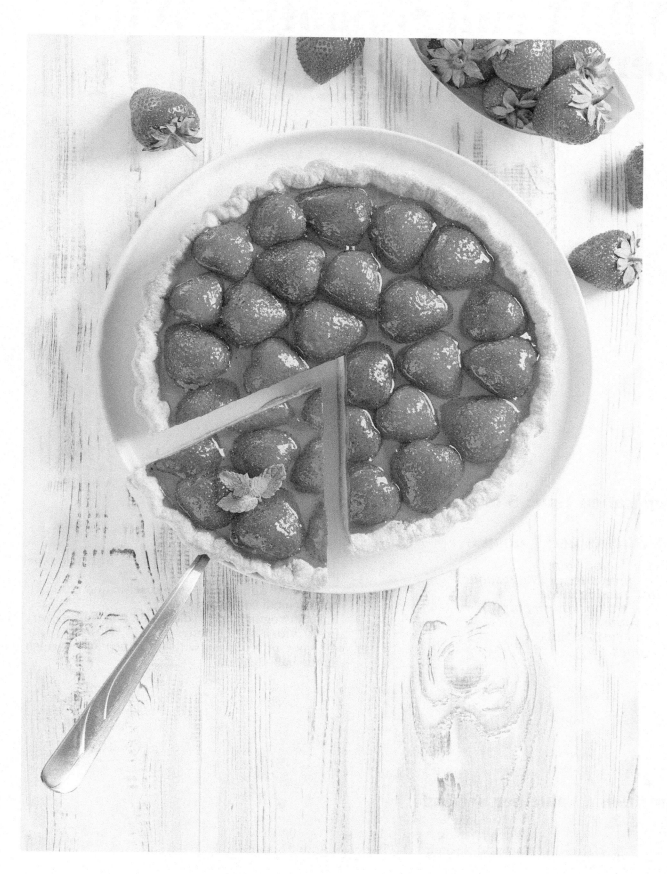

Wild Fruit Smoothie With Lemon Balm

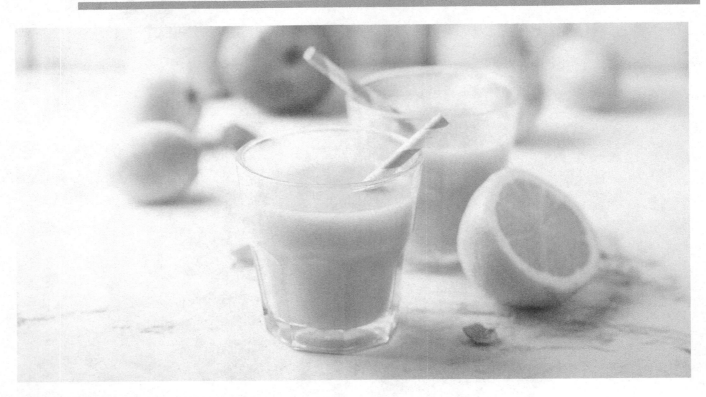

Preparation Time: 5 min

Ingredients per 1 people

- *1 stem lemon balm*
- *50 g applesauce (without sugar)*
- *1 tbsp rosehip pulp*
- *1 tbsp sea buckthorn pulp*
- *50 g yogurt (1.5% fat)*
- *100 ml curdled milk*
- *ice cubes*

1. Rinse the lemon balm, shake dry and pluck the leaves off.
2. Put the applesauce with rosehip and sea buckthorn pulp in a tall container.
3. Add yogurt and curdled milk and puree everything finely with a hand blender.
4. Pour into a glass with ice cubes and garnish with lemon balm leaves.

Nutritional Value per Serving

193 Kcal	7g Fat	22g Carbs	8g Protein	1g Fiber	0g Added Sugar

Banana Berry Smoothie with Grapefruit

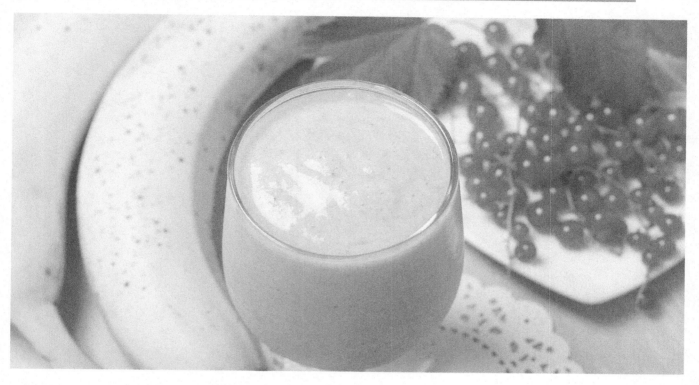

Preparation Time: 10 min

Ingredients for 2 people:

- *300 g grapefruit (1 grapefruit)*
- *300 g ripe bananas (2 ripe bananas)*
- *500 g red currants*
- *1 tsp barley grass (powder)*
- *ice cubes*

1. Halve the grapefruit, squeeze it and put the juice in a blender.
2. Peel the bananas, cut the pulp into slices and also put them in the blender.
3. Wash the currants, drain them and set aside 2 beautiful panicles.
4. Strip the rest of the berries from the panicles and put them in the blender.
5. Add the barley grass and ice cubes.
6. Mix everything well, pour into 2 glasses and garnish with the currant panicles set aside.

Nutritional Value per Serving

241 Kcal	1g Fat	46g Carbs	4g Protein	20g Fiber	0g Added Sugar

CROHN'S DISEASE RESOURCES

L iving with Crohn's disease can be a challenge that requires multiple sources of information and support. Here are some websites, articles and organizations that might be of assistance.

Organizations

Crohn's Colitis Foundation

Founded in 1967, this group promotes education, research and advocacy on Crohn's disease and ulcerative colitis.
https://www.crohnscolitisfoundation.org/

Intense Intestines Foundation

This non-profit organization aims to help patients with Crohn's disease, ulcerative colitis, and ostomies by connecting them through social media engagement and unique events.
https://www.mightycause.com/organization/Intenseintestines

Centers for Disease Control and Prevention (CDC)

This U.S. federal agency funds research and provides information on Crohn's disease, including tracking its prevalence in the United States.

https://www.cdc.gov/ibd/

American Gastroenterological Association

This leading professional organization for gastroenterologists promotes education for both doctors and patients and publishes care standards for Crohn's disease.
https://www.gastro.org/

American College of Gastroenterology

This gastroenterologists organization promotes training and education for doctors and provides information for patients on various conditions. https://gi.org/

Connecting to Cure Crohn's & Colitis

This California non-profit aspires to promote public awareness about Crohn's disease and ulcerative colitis, support patients and their families, and fund research for new treatments and cures for inflammatory bowel diseases.

https://www.connectingtocure.org/

Financial Assistance

Partnership for Prescription Assistance

This free service connects patients to many private and public assistance programs that provide financial assistance for prescription drugs.
https://medicineassistancetool.org/

NeedyMeds

This organization offers a drug discount card and resources for finding pharmacies with the lowest prices.
https://www.needymeds.org/

Social Security Administration

This federal agency provides numerous insurance and safety net programs, including disability benefits for eligible applicants.

https://www.ssa.gov/

Coping, Advocacy, and Support

Crohn's & Colits Community

The Crohn's & Colitis Foundation website contains patient stories, an online support group, a discussion forum, and an expert Q&A page.
https://www.crohnscolitiscommunity.org/

Find a Chapter — Crohn's & Colitis Foundation

This page lets you search for a local arm of this national organization near you.
https://www.crohnscolitisfoundation.org/chapters/

Advocacy Tools and Resources — Crohn's & Colitis Foundation

On this page, you can connect to a variety of materials on getting involved in this group Crohn's-related advocacy.
https://www.crohnscolitisfoundation.org/chapters/

Crohnology

This website lets patients share treatment and management strategies that have worked for them and uses a statistical approach to rate treatments.
https://crohnology.com/

Statistics and Information

Talk With an Information Specialist — Crohn's & Colitis Foundation

This page lets you connect with a specialist on Crohn's disease by email, phone, or live video chat during certain hours.
https://www.crohnscolitisfoundation.org/living-with-crohns-colitis/talk-to-a-specialist/

Data and Statistics — CDC

On this page, you can find statistics on the prevalence of Crohn's disease in the United States.
https://www.cdc.gov/ibd/data-statistics.htm

Alternative Therapies

Complementary and Alternative Medicine (CAM)

This page illustrates many alternative therapies that have been tried for Crohn's disease and how strong the evidence is for various practices.
https://www.crohnscolitisfoundation.org/resources/complementary-alternative.html

10 Alternative Therapies for Crohn's Disease

This article provides a list of alternative treatments that may be helpful in Crohn's disease.
https://www.everydayhealth.com/hs/crohns-disease-treatment-management/complementary-alternative-therapies-for-crohns/

Specialists and Treatment Facilities

Find a Healthcare Professional — Crohn's & Colitis Foundation

This page allows you to search for doctors, nurses, and other health professionals who are members of the CCF.

https://www.crohnscolitisfoundation.org/living-with-crohns-colitis/find-a-doctor/

Find a Gastroenterologist — American College of Gastroenterology

On this page, you can search for a gastroenterologist near to you who is a member of the American College of Gastroenterology.

https://patients.gi.org/find-a-gastroenterologist/

Patient and Doctor Blogs

Ali on the Run

This blog, owned by a running enthusiast with Crohn's disease living in New York City, illustrates the ups and downs of living with the condition. It also has a companion podcast.

https://www.aliontherunblog.com/

Lights, Camera, Crohn's

In Natalie Hayden's famous blog, she writes about juggling the ups and downs of life with Crohn's disease while raising two kids.

https://lightscameracrohns.com/

Own Your Crohn's

Tina Aswani Omprakash blogs about her personal experience living with Crohn's disease and all things related to inflammatory bowel disease (IBD), including culture, lifestyle, and diversity, caregiving, and clinical trials. She also interviews other patients about their experiences living with the condition.

https://ownyourcrohns.com/

The Crohn's Colitis Effect

This site contains blog posts from various people living with Crohn's disease and video interviews with patients, parents, and others affected by this condition.

https://cceffect.org/

Inflamed & Untamed

This blog describes the struggles of living as a young woman with multiple medical conditions — including Crohn's disease — and without a colon.
https://www.inflamed-and-untamed.com/

Jenni's Gut

This blog provides an account of living with Crohn's disease and fibromyalgia, anxiety, insomnia, and chronic nausea.
https://jennisguts.blogspot.com/

Crohn's Disease — Leaving the Seat Down

This is a blog of the musings and artwork of a Canadian man with Crohn's disease.
https://jennisguts.blogspot.com/

The Stolen Colon

This blog describes "living beautifully" as a young mother with Crohn's disease and an ostomy.
http://stolencolon.com/

For Children and Teens

GIKids

GIKids provides easy-to-understand information about the treatment and management of these pediatric digestive conditions for children and parents.
http://www.gikids.org/

Just Like Me Teens with IBD

Website for teens with IBD powered by the CCF. It offers information about life with Crohn's, treatments and research, as well as ways to connect with other teens with IBD, including support groups and forums.
http://www.justlikemeibd.org/z-testing/cddev/2017-just-like-me/

Nationwide Children's

This website provides a lot of IBD resources for families, as a blog and some animations to explain children everything about Crohn's disease
https://www.nationwidechildrens.org/specialties/inflammatory-bowel-disease-clinic/ibd-resources-for-families

Life Uncommon: Inflammatory Bowel Disease (IBD)

This is a video series about children and teens with IBD and the professionals who care for them at CHOP. https://www.chop.edu/health-resources/life-uncommon-inflammatory-bowel-disease-ibd

Your Child with Inflammatory Bowel Disease

This book provides parents with practical information on how to talk to their children about IBD. It also discusses challenges for children at school and in their social lives. https://www.amazon.com/Your-Child-Inflammatory-Bowel-Disease/dp/0801895561

Clinical Trials

Clinical Trials Community — Crohn's & Colitis Foundation

This page connects to resources on a clinical trial, how it might help you, and how to find trials you might be eligible for.
https://www.crohnscolitisfoundation.org/clinical-trials-community

ClinicalTrials.gov

This website offers a searchable database of clinical trials nationwide, including those related to Crohn's disease.
https://clinicaltrials.gov/

CenterWatch

This publisher supplies information about clinical trials in a variety of formats to both doctors and patients.
https://www.centerwatch.com/

What Did You Think of "The New Crohn's Friendly Cookbook"?

First of all, thank you for purchasing The New Crohn's Friendly Cookbook. I know you could have picked any number of books to read, but you picked this book, and I am incredibly grateful for that.

If you enjoyed this book and found some benefit in reading this, I'd like to hear from you and hope that you could take some time to post a review on Amazon. Your feedback and support will mean a lot to me and will help me significantly for future projects.

Thanks!

Customer Reviews

⭐⭐⭐⭐⭐ 38
4.8 out of 5 stars ▾

5 star	▓▓▓▓▓▓▓	87%
4 star	▓	10%
3 star		3%
2 star		0%
1 star		0%

Share your thoughts with other customers

Write a customer review

See all 38 customer reviews ›

About the author

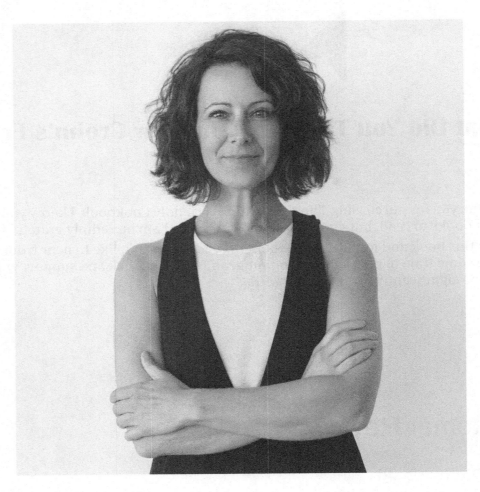

Lydia Merrill is a Certified Dietician and Nutritionist who has been counseling individuals on sustainable weight management and disease prevention for over 20 years. Her mission is to inspire individuals to obtain healthy food relationships and to clearly understand the idea of food as medicine. Lydia has a great passion for promoting easy-to-understand nutrition and diet tips and started blogging in 2017 to promote healthy eating messages in a readable and accessible manner.

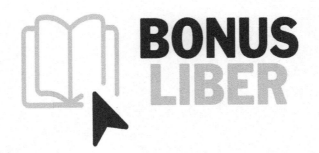